PALEO 25

Jump Start Your Healthy Eating with 25 Days of Delicious Meals

Includes Over 75 Gluten-Free, Grain-Free, Dairy-Free Recipes

No Sugar or Salt Added

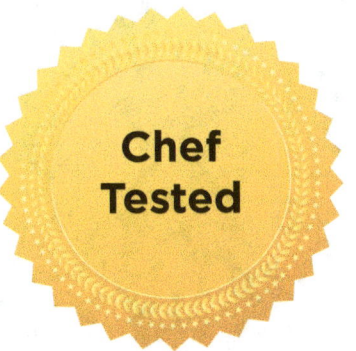

By Donna Leahy
Photography by Robert Leahy

*PALEO 25: Jump Start Your Healthy Eating
with 25 Days of Delicious Meals*

Food Arts Fusion LLC

ISBN: 978-1-942118-12-1

© 2015, Donna Leahy

ALL RIGHTS RESERVED. Any unauthorized reprint or use of this material is prohibited. No part of this book may be reproduced or transmitted in any form or by any means, electronic or mechanical, including photocopying, recording or by any information storage and retrieval system without the written permission of the author, except where permitted by law.

Disclaimer

The information contained in this book is based on research and personal experience unless otherwise stated. It should not be substituted for qualified medical advice. Health-related information provided in this book is for educational and entertainment purposes only. Always seek the counsel of a qualified medical practitioner for an individual consultation before making any significant changes to your diet and lifestyle, and to answer questions about specific medical conditions. The author and publisher disclaim responsibility for any adverse effects that may result from the use or application of the recipes and information within this book. The publisher and the author make no representations or warranties with respect to accuracy or completeness of the contents of this work and specifically disclaim all warranties including, without limitation, warranties of fitness, health or weight loss for a particular purpose. This work is sold with the understanding that the publisher and author are not engaged in rendering medical or other professional advice, and neither is liable for damages arising from it.

Also by Donna Leahy

Paleo for Weight Loss: The 14-Day Healthy Eating Plan

Paleo Easy As 1-2-3: Lose Weight, Eat Great

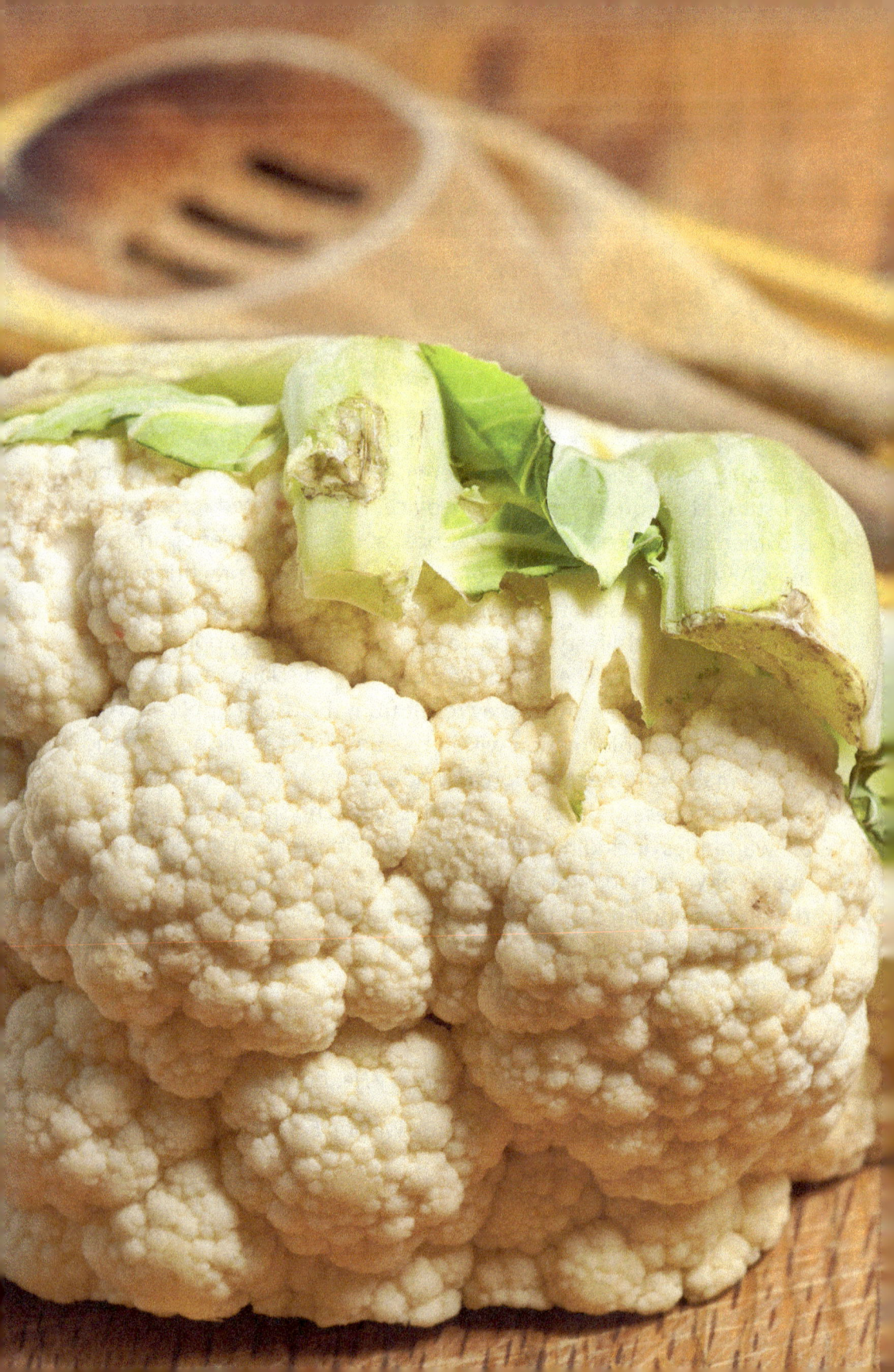

Thank you for purchasing this book. I am pleased to have you along for the journey to better health and better eating. I know you could have picked from dozens of cookbooks about Paleo, so to show my appreciation, I'd like to offer you a bonus: *PALEO 25 – TEN TERRIFIC SNACK RECIPES*. Simply sign up on my website www.donnaleahy.com and I will send you the PDF. I will include you on my list for free stuff and also periodically send you any exclusive special offerings. As an experienced chef and author, I write cookbooks on a variety of topics and themes. So even if you find Paleo is not the right eating plan for you, my other cookbooks may interest you as well.

If you have a moment to post a review of this book, I'd really appreciate it. This type of feedback will help me continue to write the kind of cookbooks that you want to use.

Thanks again, I look forward to hearing from you.

Chef Donna

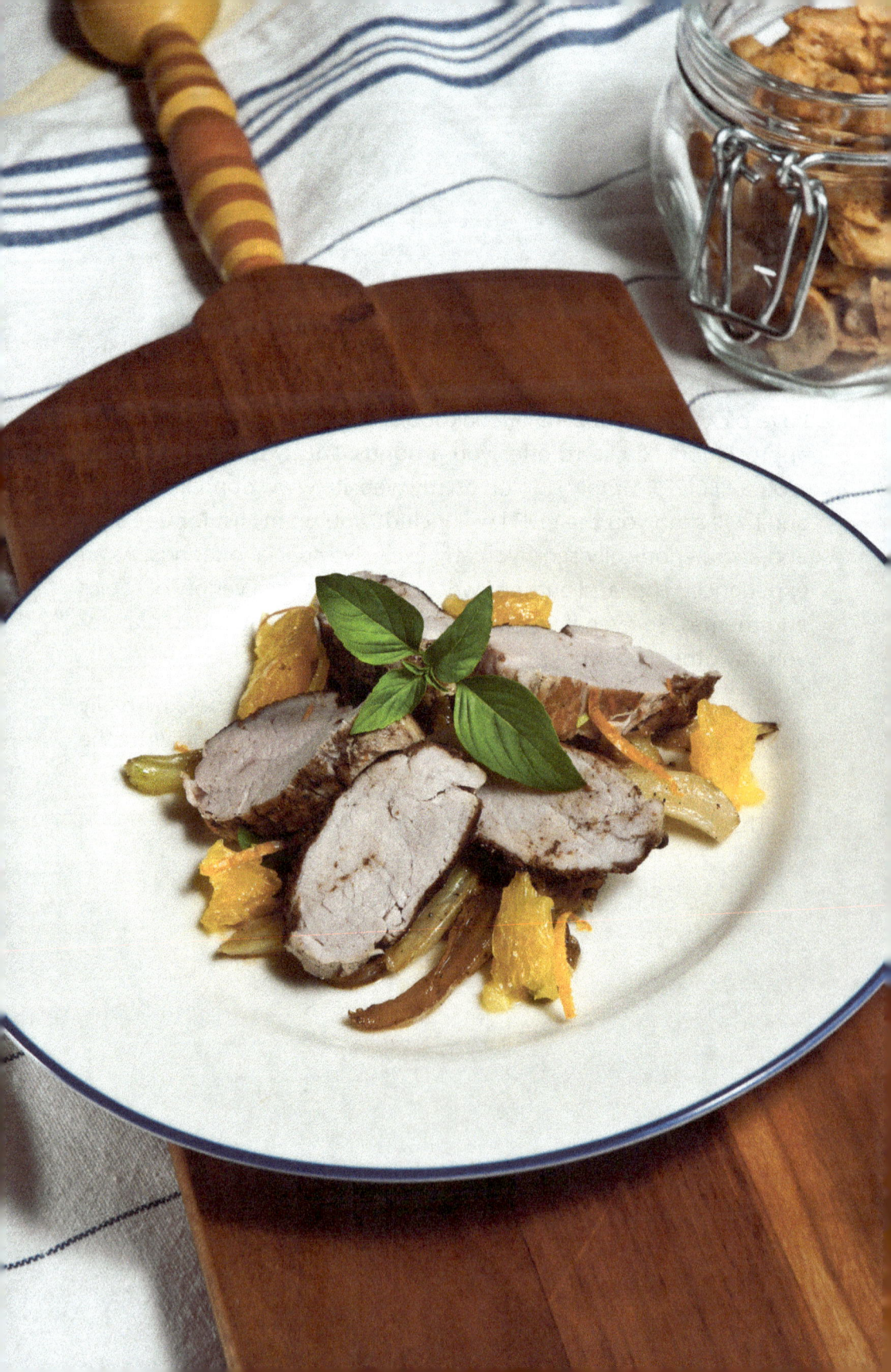

Table of Contents

Introduction 13

CHAPTER ONE
25 Breakfasts 21

Steak, Pepper and Egg with Arugula Pesto 25
Andouille-Stuffed Tomato 27
Shrimp and Dill Egg Custard 29
Salmon, Egg and Sweet Potato Pancake 31
Tuna with Poached Egg and Cherry Tomato Salsa 33
Salmon, Avocado and Pistachio Wraps 35
Eggs Lobster Oscar with Cauliflower 37
Hard-Cooked Eggs with Crab, Avocado and Belgian Endive .. 39
Salmon Deviled Eggs 41
Pork and Mango Omelet 43
Sweet Potato Skin with Spinach and Italian Sausage 45
Portobello, Sausage and Egg Stack 47
Asparagus, Egg and Tomato Tart 49
Italian Fried Eggs with Sausage and Peppers 50
Pumpkin, Pecan and Coconut Breakfast Bowl 51
Blueberry Almond Custard 53
Coddled Egg with Sun-Dried Tomatoes and Mushrooms 55
Baked Tomato with Caramelized Onions and Egg 56
Swiss Chard, Pork Belly and Bell Pepper Frittata 57
Roasted Eggplant and Cherry Tomatoes with Egg 59
Scrambled Egg Soup with Spinach 61

Bok Choy, Carrot and Radish Omelet Soup 62

Five Spice Chicken and Egg Scramble 63

Turkey, Cauliflower and Apple Soup 65

Sweet Potato Hash with Turkey and Egg 67

CHAPTER TWO
25 Lunches 69

Veal Scallops with Cherry Tomatoes and Celery 71

Steak with Mango, Arugula and Pistachios 72

Beef Short-Rib and Vegetable Soup 73

Tuna Filet with Saffron Slaw 75

Seafood and Butternut Squash Chowder 76

Chilled Cucumber, Avocado and Shrimp Soup 79

Shrimp, Red Pepper and Almond Soup 81

Seafood and Avocado Salad 83

Crab, Fennel and Asparagus Salad 84

Shrimp Papaya Salad with Cashews 85

Roasted Beet with Salmon, Walnuts and Mint 87

Pork Tenderloin with Spinach, Orange and Onions 89

Watermelon, Cucumber and Red Onion with Pork 91

Celery Root, Leek and Pork Belly Soup 92

Spicy Chicken Salad with Mustard Greens 93

Cabbage, Carrot and Apple Slaw with Chicken 95

Chicken Salad with Carrot, Radish and Cucumber 97

Spaghetti Squash Primavera with Chicken 98

Chicken and Coconut Soup with Cauliflower 101

Turkey with Roasted Sweet Potato, Turnip and Pear 103

Watercress and Sweet Potato Soup 105

Curried Zucchini Spinach Soup 106

Wild Mushroom Soup 107

Roasted Eggplant and Tomato Soup 109

Spicy Sweet Potato and Parsnip Soup 110

CHAPTER THREE
25 Dinners 111

Spicy Lamb Burger with Orange Herb Slaw 115

Lamb Tagine with Star Anise 116

Meatloaf with Roasted Red Pepper and Cauliflower 117

Filet Mignon with Celery Root and Mushrooms 120

Veal Chop with Broccoli Rabe 122

Chili and Mint Fish Cake with Broccoli Puree 125

Sesame Shrimp with Orange and Almonds 127

Lobster with Arugula and Spaghetti Squash 129

Sea Scallops with Cherry Tomatoes, Avocado
and Macadamias 131

Pan-Seared Tuna with Caramelized Onions and
Mango Salsa 133

Moroccan Fish Stew 134

Trout with Carrot and Walnuts 135

Mediterranean Halibut in Parchment 137

Salmon with Red Cabbage, Brussels Sprouts
and Hazelnuts 139

Pan-Roasted Mussels with Onions and Basil 140

Red Snapper with Leeks and Saffron 141

Pork Ribs with Jicama Slaw 143

Pork Loin Chop with Peaches, Squash and Pecans 144

Pork Tenderloin with Cherries and Kale 145

Five Spice Chicken with Tangerine and Fennel 146

Green Coconut Curry with Chicken and Cabbage 147

Chicken with Pesto and Cauliflower Puree 149

Zucchini-Stuffed Game Hen with Turnip and Mushrooms 150

Beet and Parsnip Chips with Shredded Chicken......................... 152

Turkey, Zucchini and Butternut Squash Strata 155

CHAPTER FOUR
Pantry 159

Plantain Wraps 160

Moroccan Spice Blend... 161

Chili Powder 162

Mayonnaise 163

Barbecue Sauce 164

Basil Pesto 165

Chicken Stock 166

Beef Stock 168

Fish Stock 170

Vegetable Stock... 172

Sausage... 173

Pork Belly.. 177

Appendix: Shopping List and 25 Menus 179

Index 190

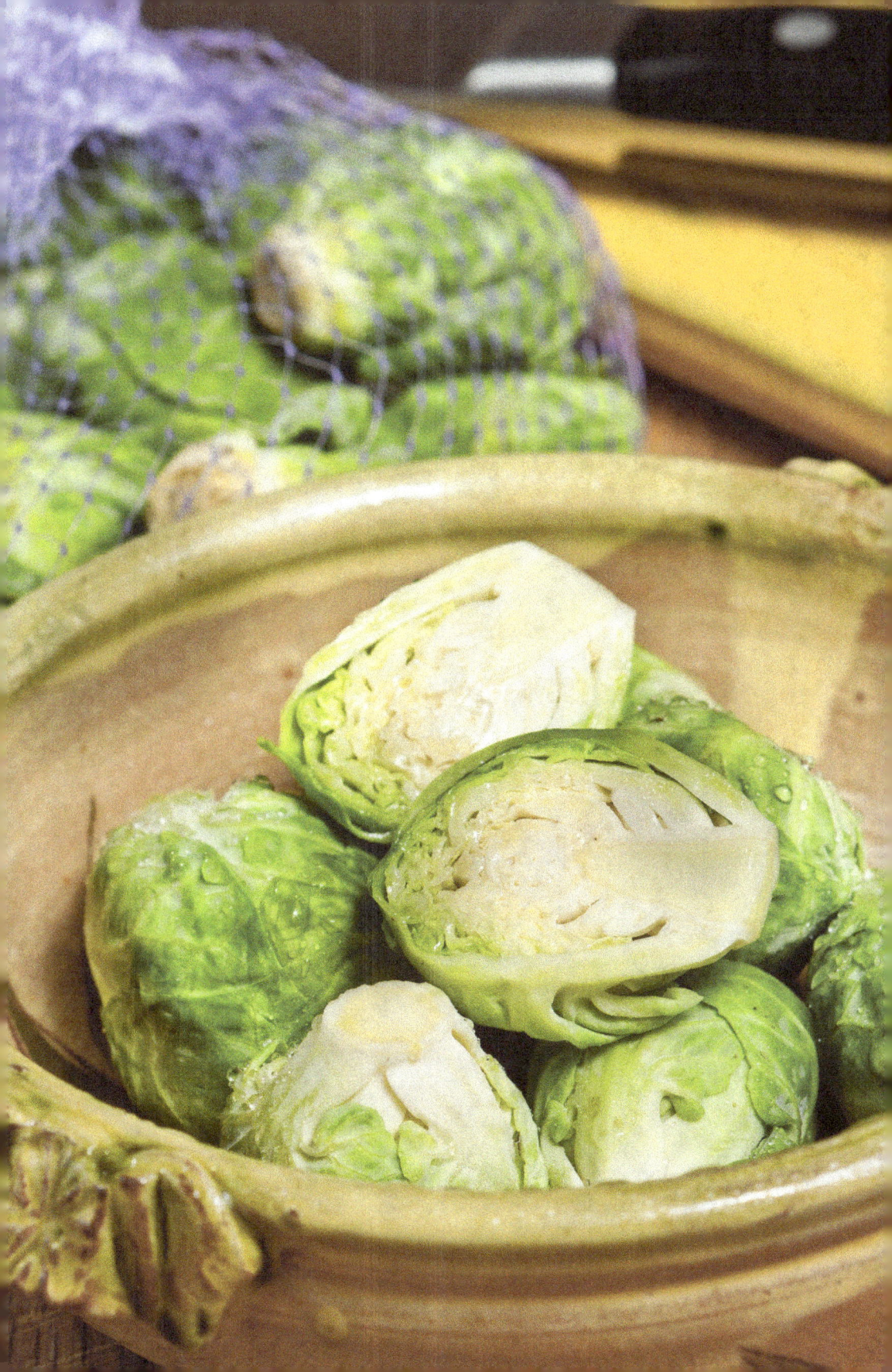

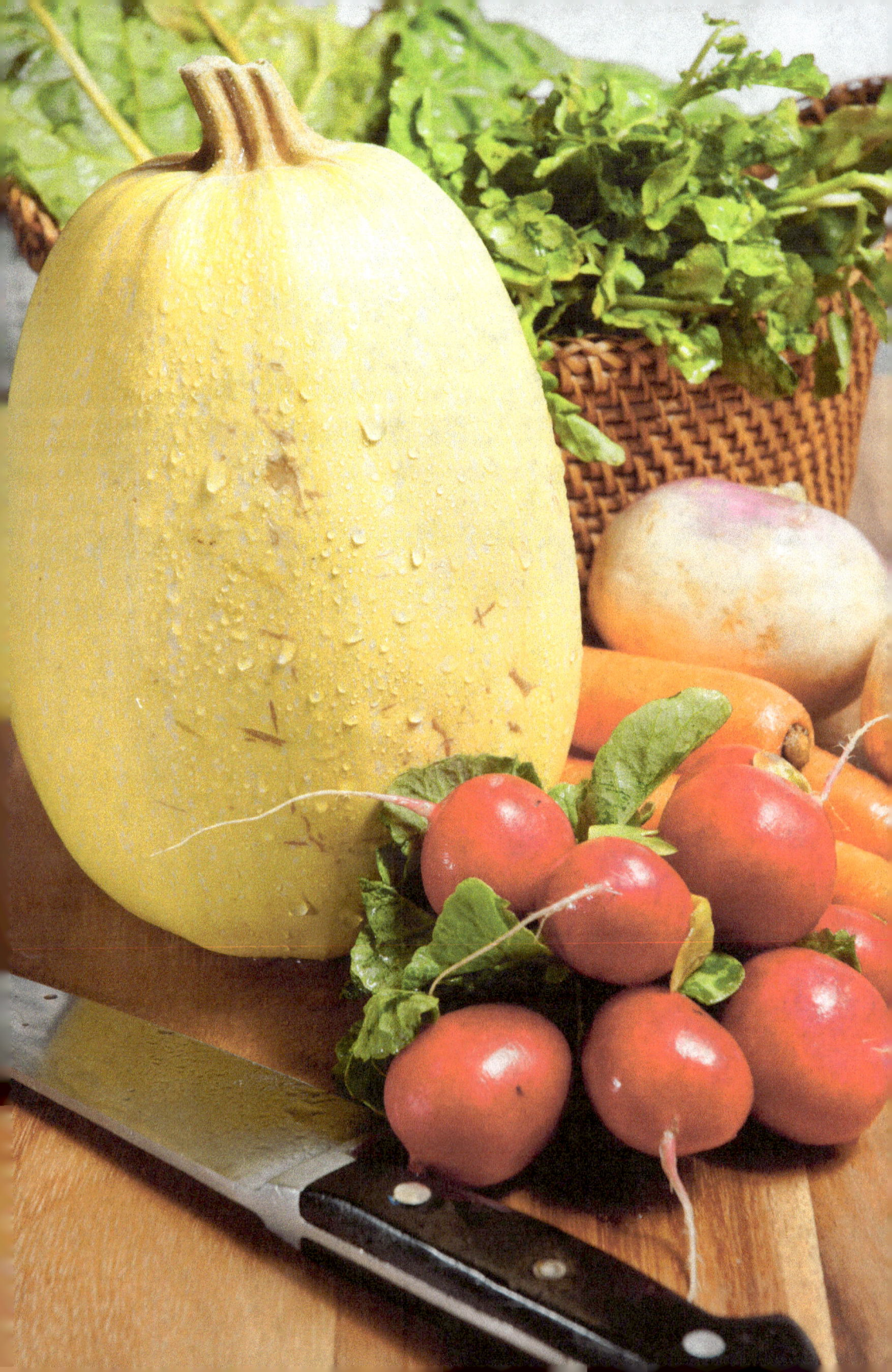

Paleo 25 Introduction

Whether you're new to Paleo or a seasoned Paleo follower, you've come to the right place. You're about to jump start your Paleo routine with 25 days of delicious, easy-to-make recipes for breakfast, lunch and dinner. If you're just starting Paleo, this book will get you on the path to losing weight and eating healthier. If you're already following Paleo, this book will become a go-to resource for original, restaurant-quality Paleo recipes for every meal of the day. If you want to use Paleo to reset your eating habits, these recipes will help you get there while enjoying great food.

Unlike other books that repeat recipes found online or provide "Paleo-ized" versions of well-known dishes, these recipes are all originals, based on a strict interpretation of Paleo without compromising taste. Please don't let the word "strict" scare you off. As a professional chef, I am acutely aware that, in order to enjoy eating, food needs to taste good. As someone who has tried every healthy eating diet on the planet, I also understand that sticking with a plan is easier if you enjoy what you are eating. The recipes to follow are proof that you can enjoy tasty meals that are easy to prepare while keeping with the Paleo lifestyle. If you want to eat healthier, lose weight or simply add variety to your current routine, these great-tasting recipes provide an easy-to-follow roadmap.

You may have heard Paleo referred to as the "Caveman Diet" or "Prehistoric Diet." But the idea of eating better goes far beyond copying the diet of our ancestors. Following Paleo helps reset what our bodies crave by eliminating the main source of trouble—our reliance on processed food. If we stop eating processed food, we stop craving it. It also eliminates some food groups that can cause our blood sugar to bounce up and down like a Ping-Pong ball. Getting that blood sugar in a stable and healthy range is the long-term approach to ending unhealthy cravings.

Understanding the guidelines to Paleo is just the first step to following the plan. Any road to healthier eating can get bumpy if we feel that we're limiting taste by limiting choices. The recipes that follow are designed to help you stay on the Paleo path, with some exciting ways of preparing meals for any time of the day. Of course, it's up to you to decide how you will incorporate Paleo into your lifestyle and to choose when, if ever, you deviate from the plan. But if you want to use the plan to feel healthier and lose the cravings, there are several benefits of adhering to the approach followed in this book.

First, if you've tried Paleo and aren't having good results, you may be sabotaging yourself by following recipes that don't really stick with the plan—especially if you are new to Paleo. There are a lot of recipes labeled as Paleo in books and online that simply don't follow the guidelines. *Paleo 25* features recipes that clearly utilize only those ingredients included in the Paleo plan. If you believe that the reasoning behind following Paleo is compelling, or are simply using it to reset eating habits, then opting in and out of certain facets of the plan may be keeping you from succeeding. As the saying goes, the idea here is to talk the talk *and* walk the walk.

Second, if you are using Paleo to reset your eating habits and reduce cravings, it is important that you pay attention to how your food is being prepared and understand why certain ingredients are off the list. For example, recipes that include cured meat like bacon, salami or prosciutto miss the point that all of these items are 1) processed food and 2) salt-cured (i.e., high in added salt), which conflicts with basic tenets of the plan. Adding so-called "natural" sugars like maple syrup, honey and agave nectar also contradicts one of main components of the plan (i.e., eliminating added sugar). Creating Paleo baked goods like muffins, pancakes and bread also undermines the idea of reducing cravings for these items by eliminating them altogether.

Creating replacement items for processed foods (have you been searching for Paleo bread at the natural foods grocery?) misses the point that eliminating them benefits your personal health.

Third, once you've tried the Paleo plan as it was originally intended, it's up to you when and how you might deviate from it. After resetting your eating habits, you will be empowered to decide what works for you. If you do choose to deviate from the original plan, you will decide how you feel after adding any particular food. Being mindful about what we eat is one of the most important tenets of Paleo. It's an important concept that cuts across all dietary plans in that it begins with you making conscious choices about what you consume. Following the Paleo plan in this manner gives you a framework to rethink and reevaluate what you eat, one meal at a time.

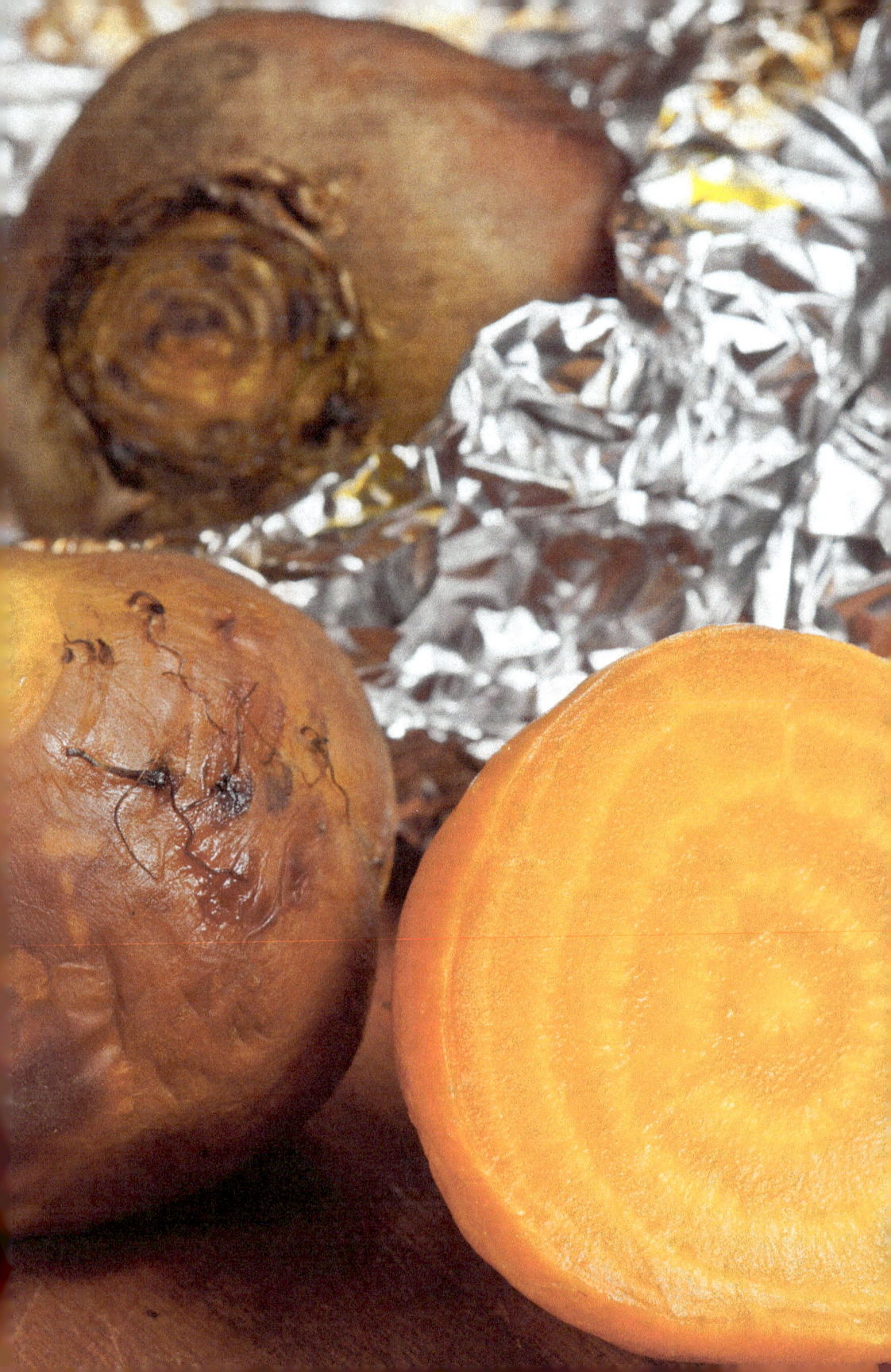

About the Recipes

All of the recipes for breakfast, lunch and dinner are developed to serve one person. This makes it easy for you to cook for yourself or to increase the number of portions to serve additional people. Because the meals taste delicious, it will be easy to get your family members or partner to enjoy them without actually feeling they are being restricted in any way. They are developed to enjoy alone but are also perfect for entertaining.

What you won't find in this book are basic recipes like how to grill a steak, roast a chicken or toss a green salad. If you've been following Paleo for a while, I am guessing you're also a pro at converting taco recipes to lettuce wraps, making spaghetti squash with meatballs and perhaps even preparing chia protein shakes. The goal is to offer both the beginner and the experienced Paleo follower something new and unique. These dishes will up your cooking game and keep you interested in following Paleo. Included are 75 original, inventive, step-by-step recipes for preparing delicious Paleo meals, plus a bonus chapter with recipes for pantry items. In the Appendix, you'll find a detailed shopping list and 25 days of menus incorporating all of the recipes.

In addition to not finding recipes for basic dishes in this book, you will also not find Paleo versions of baked treats, including cookies, cake, pancakes or waffles. It's hard to justify using 90 almonds in a cup of almond flour to make a recipe for a muffin, or adding sugar to it under the guise of it being "natural," especially if you are trying to lose weight and reduce cravings. (Of course, almond flour may be used in moderation on Paleo.) There is also no added salt in any of the recipes.

There are suggestions about when to make extra protein at dinner so you'll have some easy options available when it comes to preparing other meals. Some of the breakfast and lunch recipes are written without meat or seafood, giving you the option to add them according to your personal preference. Somehow Paleo is often associated with a meat eater's dream, akin to Atkins and other high-protein diets. But in the original Paleo plan, 30–35% of caloric intake is derived from protein (from many different sources that include meat), 30% comes from fats and 40% comes from carbohydrates—in other words, you need to eat your veggies (and a little fruit) too.

Finally, these recipes were developed and tested as restaurant-quality dishes, so the various elements of the dish are intended to enhance each other. I hope you'll enjoy the interesting combination of texture and flavor inherent in each dish. However, I've also made recommendations for substitutions or additions in case there is an ingredient you don't personally enjoy. There are 25 recipes for each meal of the day that can be followed for consecutive days for weight loss or to reduce cravings, or inserted into your current Paleo eating routine if you are simply seeking more variety. No matter how you incorporate the recipes, you will be enjoying delicious new Paleo meals that are easy to prepare.

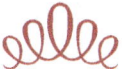

A Quick Review of Paleo

As a brief recap, here is a list of what's not included in the recipes to follow:

- Grains, including pseudo-grains like quinoa
- Legumes, including beans, peas and peanuts
- Added salt in all forms, including cured meats like bacon
- Refined vegetable oils including soybean, canola, peanut and corn oil
- Vinegars and other fermented foods, like fish sauce
- Soy
- Added sugar in all forms, including honey
- Dairy
- White potatoes

Cooking your own food is the most important first step you can make towards improving your health. Making thoughtful choices about how your ingredients are farmed and raised will also go a long way to improving your enjoyment of food. In the Appendix, you will find a detailed shopping list for the recipes in this book. This list will give you an idea of the great variety of delicious foods you will be consuming. Since the emphasis of this book is on cooking great-tasting healthy food (and not a guide to the "why" of Paleo), let's get straight to the recipes.

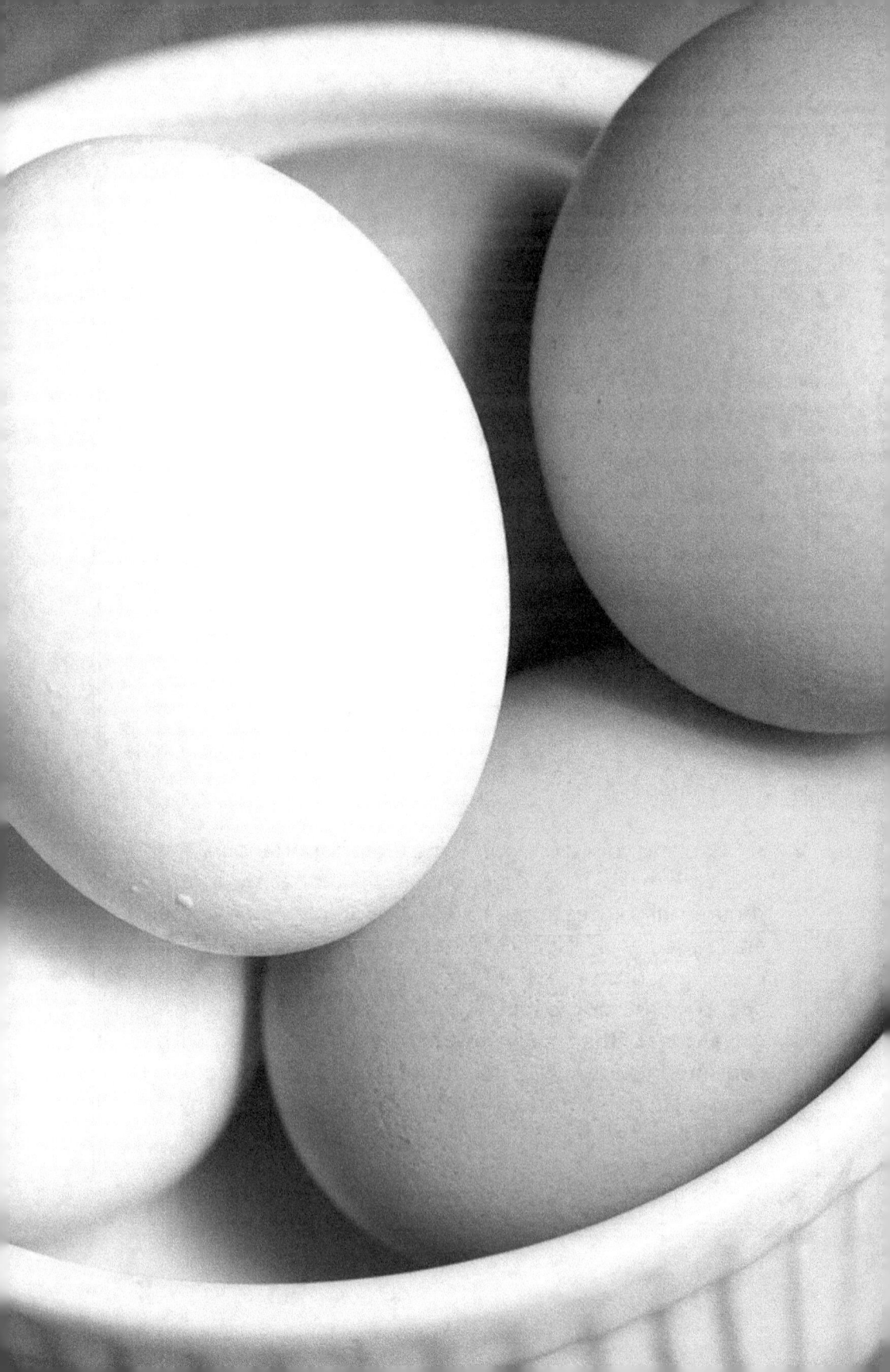

CHAPTER ONE

25 Breakfasts

- Steak, Pepper and Egg with Arugula Pesto
- Shrimp and Dill Egg Custard
- Salmon, Egg and Sweet Potato Pancake
- Tuna with Poached Egg and Cherry Tomato Salsa
- Salmon, Avocado and Pistachio Wraps
- Eggs Lobster Oscar with Cauliflower
- Hard-Cooked Eggs with Crab, Avocado and Belgian Endive
- Salmon Deviled Eggs
- Pork and Mango Omelet
- Sweet Potato Skin with Spinach and Italian Sausage
- Portobello, Sausage and Egg Stack
- Andouille-Stuffed Tomato
- Italian Fried Eggs with Sausage and Peppers
- Asparagus, Egg and Tomato Tart
- Pumpkin, Pecan and Coconut Breakfast Bowl
- Blueberry Almond Custard
- Baked Tomato with Caramelized Onions and Egg
- Coddled Egg with Sun-Dried Tomatoes and Mushrooms
- Swiss Chard and Bell Pepper Frittata
- Roasted Eggplant and Cherry Tomatoes with Egg

- Bok Choy, Carrot and Radish Omelet Soup
- Scrambled Egg Soup with Spinach
- Turkey, Cauliflower and Apple Soup
- Five Spice Chicken and Egg Scramble
- Sweet Potato Hash with Turkey and Egg

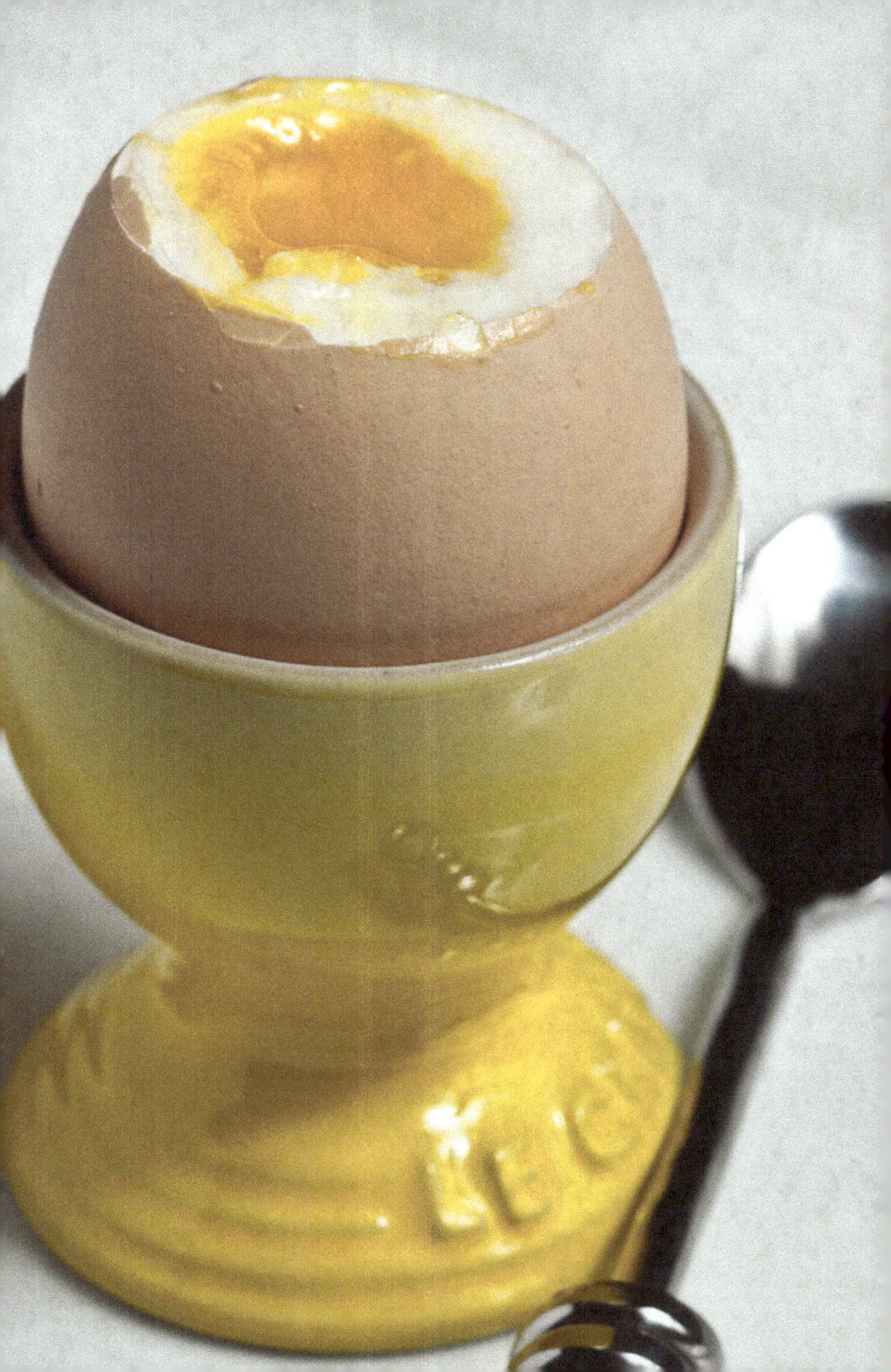

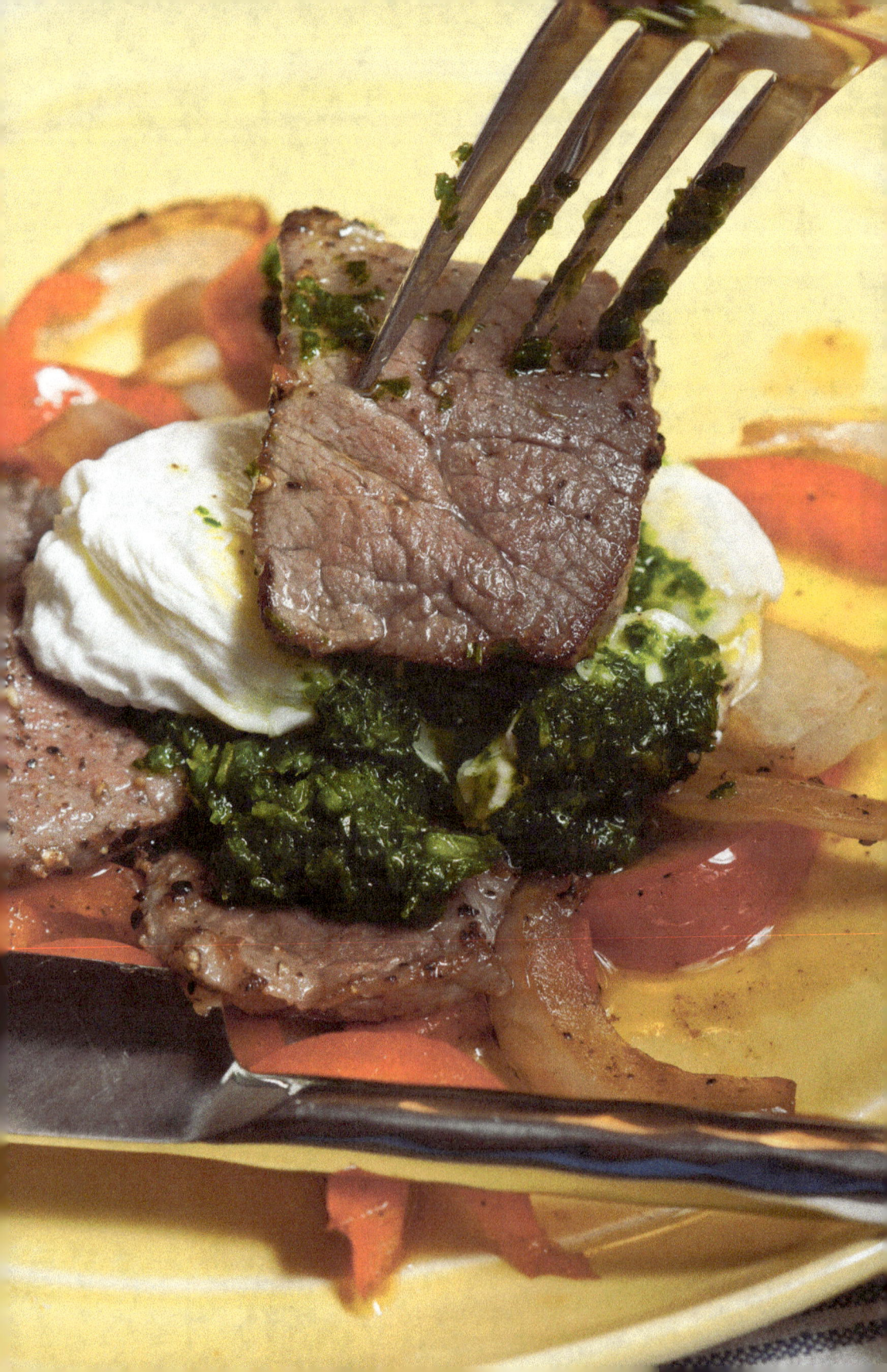

Steak, Pepper and Egg with Arugula Pesto

The classic breakfast combination of steak and eggs gets an update with a savory arugula pesto. The pesto includes pecans for texture but tastes delicious without them as well.

SERVES 1

- ¼ tsp. minced garlic
- 1 cup packed arugula leaves (about 1 oz.)
- 8 pecans (optional)
- 3 tbsps. extra virgin olive oil
- ½ tsp. lemon juice
- 3 oz. thinly sliced beef tenderloin
- ⅛ sweet onion, peeled and thinly sliced
- ¼ red bell pepper, seeded and thinly sliced
- 1–2 large eggs

In a food processor, combine the garlic, arugula and pecans (if using) and process until smooth. With the machine running, drizzle in 2 ½ tbsps. olive oil and process until smooth, scraping down the sides of the bowl as needed. Stir in the lemon juice and season with freshly ground pepper to taste. Set aside.

Heat the remaining ½ tbsp. olive oil in a small skillet over medium-high heat. Season the steak with freshly ground pepper. Sear the steak until lightly browned, about 1 minute per side. Remove from the pan and cover to keep warm. Add the onion to the pan and cook until softened, about 4–5 minutes. Add the pepper and sauté until just softened and lightly browned, about 4–5 minutes longer. Remove from the heat and keep warm.

To poach the eggs, fill a medium, deep skillet with about 2 ½" of water and bring the water to a boil. Lower the heat until the water is at a gentle simmer. Take a spoon and swirl it around the inner edge of the pan a few times to create a whirlpool effect. Immediately crack the egg and then hold it very close to the water to allow it to slip in gently.

Slide a slotted spoon under the egg to keep it from sticking to the bottom and to collect the egg white into a ball around the yolk. (Add the second egg if serving and repeat the process.) Cover the pan and simmer the egg for 3–5 minutes, until the whites are set and depending on how runny you like the yolk. Remove the egg with a slotted spoon and blot with a paper towel.

Spoon the pepper and onion mixture onto a plate. Layer on the steak slices and place the poached egg on top. Drizzle on the arugula pesto to serve.

Andouille-Stuffed Tomato

This delicious, easy-to-prepare morning meal is a tasty alternative to eggs. The sausage filling is studded with zucchini and topped with lime-scented avocado. Substitute chorizo or Italian sausage according to taste.

SERVES 1

- 1 tsp. extra virgin olive oil
- 1 tbsp. chopped onion
- 3 oz. Andouille sausage, crumbled (see recipe p. 173)
- ¼ medium zucchini, peeled and diced
- 1 tsp. chopped fresh thyme
- 1 tbsp. chopped walnuts
- 1 medium slicing tomato, cored
- 1 tbsp. chopped avocado
- 1 tsp. lime juice
- 1 tsp. chopped cilantro

Preheat the oven to 400 degrees F. Lightly grease a small baking dish or rimmed baking sheet.

Heat the olive oil in a small skillet over medium-high heat. Add the onion and cook until softened, about 4–5 minutes. Add the sausage and sauté until just cooked through, about 3–4 minutes. Add the zucchini and stir for 1 minute. Remove from the heat and stir in the thyme and walnuts.

Place the tomato into the baking dish. Spoon the mixture into the tomato. Bake for 12–15 minutes, until the tomato is softened. Combine the avocado, lime juice and cilantro in a small bowl. Spoon the avocado mixture onto the tomato and season with freshly ground pepper to serve.

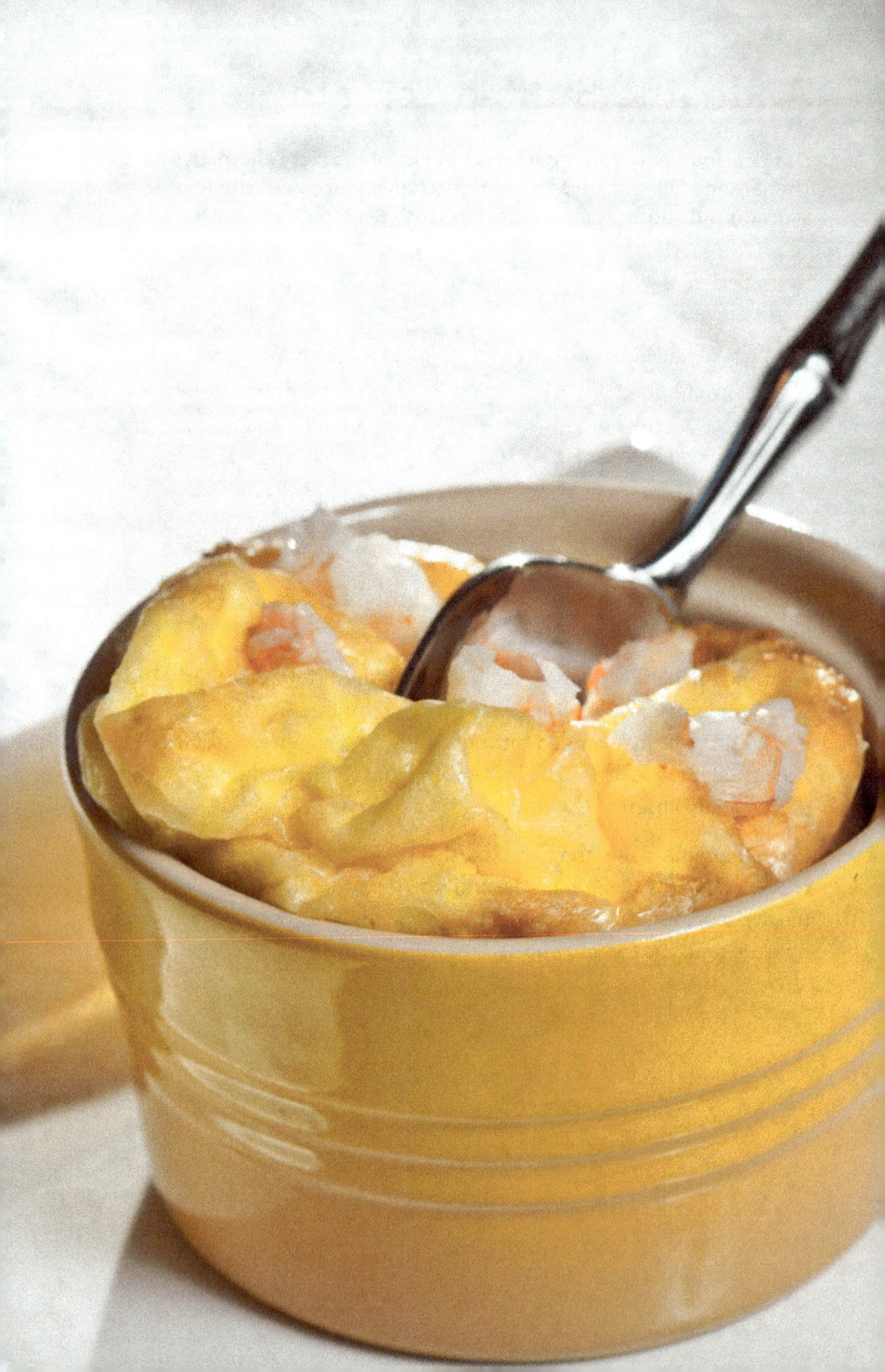

Shrimp and Dill Egg Custard

Similar to a crust-less quiche, this easy-to-assemble custard bakes in less than 20 minutes.

SERVES 1

- 2 large eggs
- 3 tbsps. coconut milk
- 1 tsp. chopped fresh dill
- 7–8 large (31–35 per lb.) cooked shrimp, coarsely chopped

Preheat oven to 350 degrees F. Lightly grease an individual ramekin.

In a medium bowl, whisk the eggs, coconut milk and dill together and season the mixture with freshly ground pepper to taste. Fill the ramekin halfway up with the egg mixture. Add the shrimp. Pour the remaining egg mixture over the top. Bake for 15–20 minutes, until mixture is set and top is puffed and lightly browned. Remove from the oven and serve immediately.

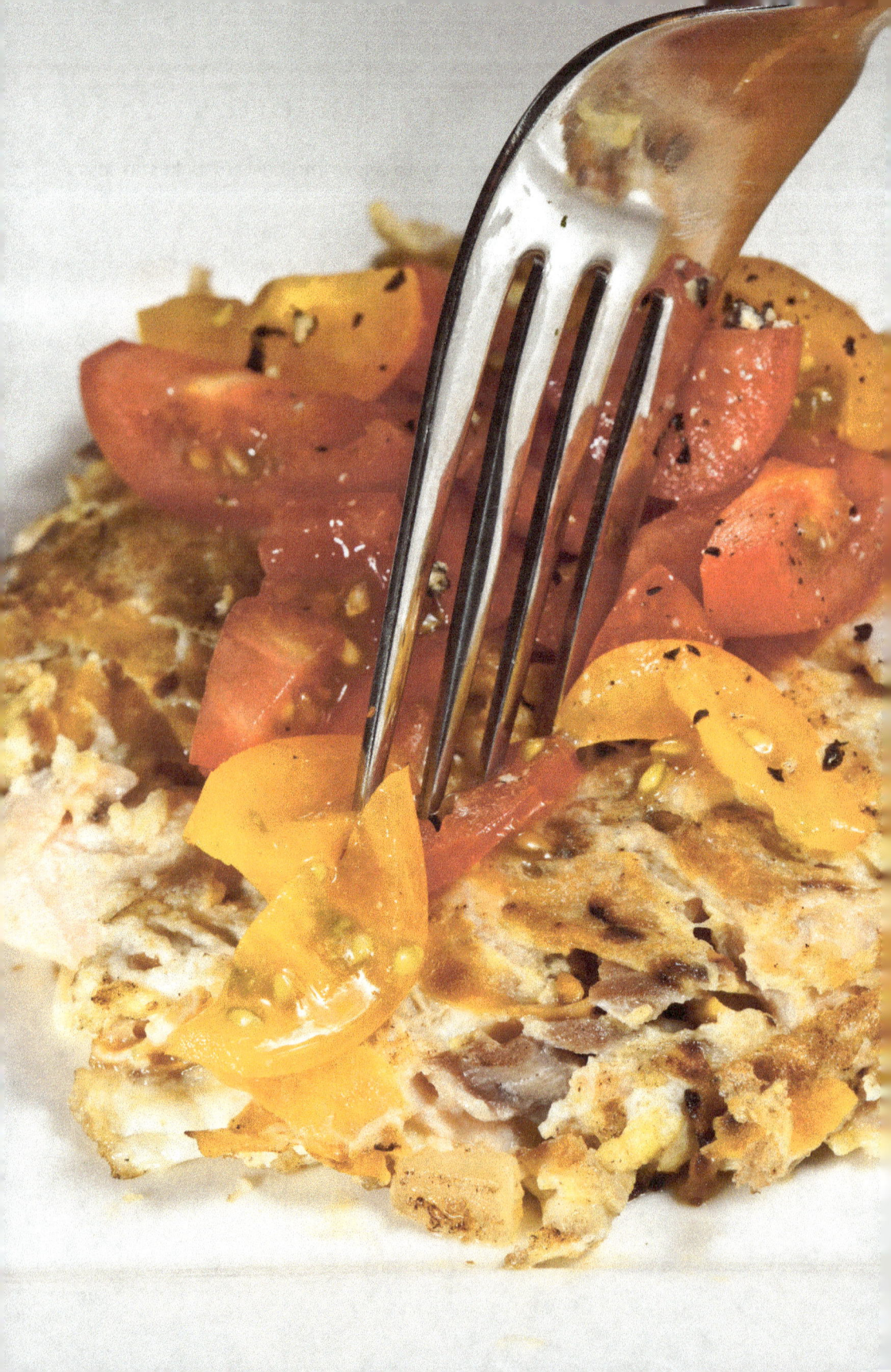

Salmon, Egg and Sweet Potato Pancake

Heart-healthy salmon and egg are blended with shredded sweet potato for a delicious savory breakfast that's easy to prepare.

SERVES 1

- 1 large egg
- 3–4 oz. cooked salmon filet, crumbled
- Pinch dried mustard
- 1 tsp. chopped fresh dill
- 3 tsps. extra virgin olive oil
- ½ sweet potato, peeled and shredded
- 2 tbsps. chopped onion

Whisk the egg in a medium bowl. Stir in the salmon, mustard and dill and set aside.

Heat 2 tsps. oil in medium skillet over medium-high heat. Add the potato and onion to the pan. Lower the heat, cover the pan and cook for 5 minutes, stirring every minute or so to prevent sticking. Remove the lid and add the remaining 1 tsp. oil. Continue cooking and stirring until the potatoes are slightly crisp and browned, about 3–4 minutes longer. Stir in the salmon egg mixture. Allow the eggs to begin to set up, then use a spatula to form the mixture into a patty about 4" in diameter. Cook for 2 minutes, then turn the patty and cook for 1–2 minutes longer, until the egg is just cooked through. Season with pepper to serve.

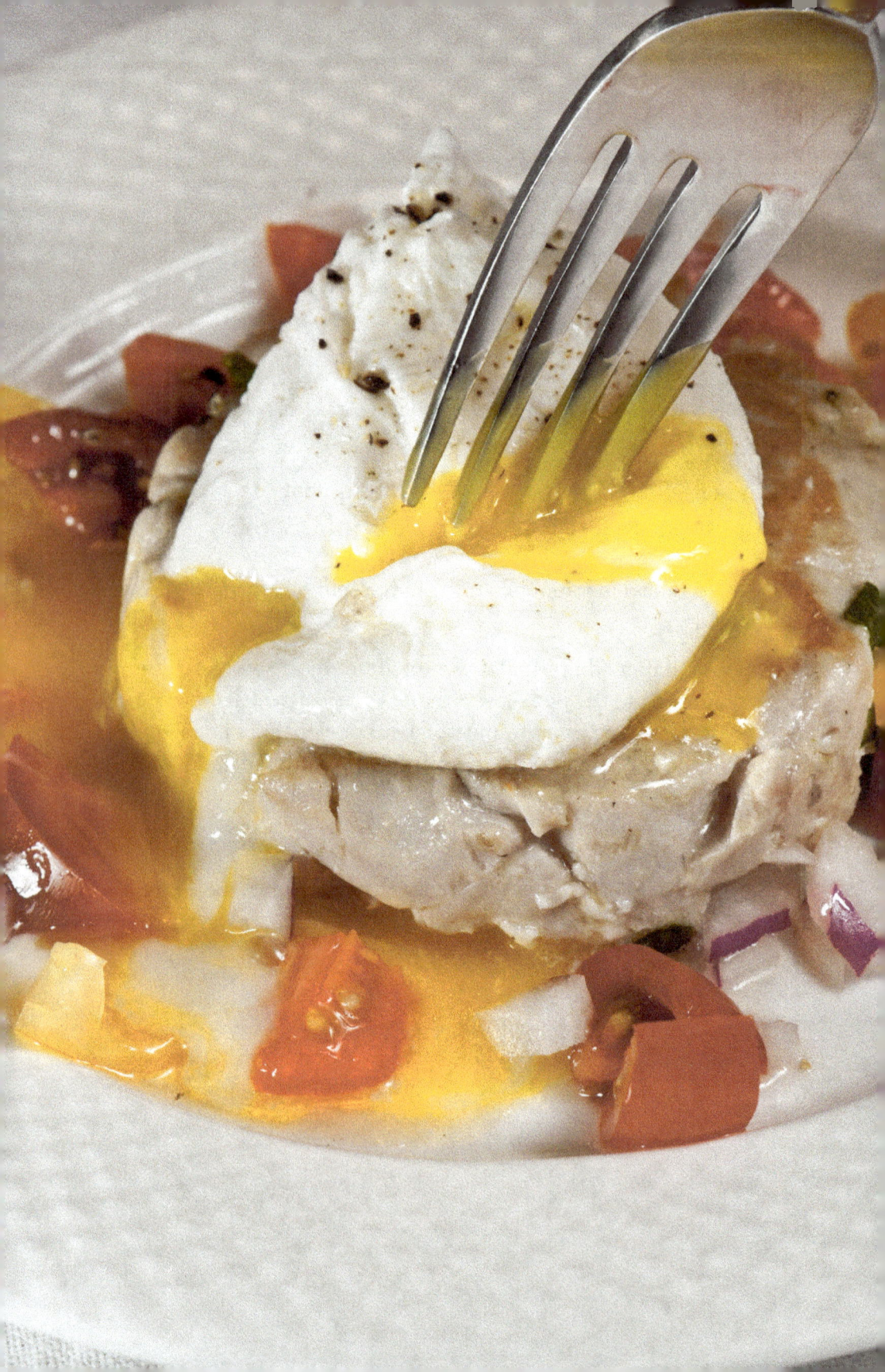

Tuna with Poached Egg and Cherry Tomato Salsa

This fresh tuna patty is flavored with grated horseradish for an added kick (or substitute a pinch of dry wasabi) and topped with a cool, refreshing salsa. The poached egg adds an elegant flair, but this breakfast dish is also delicious served with an egg cooked to your choosing (or without the egg for an even simpler preparation).

SERVES 1

- 3 tsps. extra virgin olive oil
- 1 tsp. lemon juice
- ¼ tsp. minced garlic
- 8 cherry tomatoes, coarsely chopped
- 1 tbsp. chopped red onion
- 4 oz. fresh tuna filet, cut into ¼" dice
- 1 tsp. chopped fresh flat-leaf parsley
- 1 tsp. mayonnaise (see recipe p. 163)
- 1 scallion, trimmed and minced
- ¼ tsp. freshly grated horseradish
- ¼ tsp. dry mustard
- 1–2 large eggs

Combine 2 tsps. olive oil, lemon juice and garlic in a small bowl. Add the tomatoes and onion and toss to combine. Season with freshly ground pepper and set aside.

Combine the tuna, parsley, mayonnaise, scallion and mustard. Shape the tuna into a 1-inch-thick patty. Wrap in plastic wrap and refrigerate for 20 minutes.

To poach the eggs, fill a medium, deep skillet with about 2 ½" of water and bring the water to a boil. Lower the heat until the water is at a gentle simmer. Take a spoon and swirl it around the inner edge of the pan a few times to create a whirlpool effect. Immediately crack the egg and then hold it very close to the water to allow it to slip in gently. Slide a slotted spoon under the egg to keep it from sticking to the bottom, and to collect the egg white into a ball around the yolk. (Add the second egg if serving and repeat the process.) Cover the pan and simmer the egg for 3–5 minutes, until the whites are set and depending on how runny you like the yolk. Remove the egg with a slotted spoon and blot it with a paper towel.

Heat the remaining 1 tsp. oil in a small skillet over medium-high heat. Add the tuna and cook until lightly browned, about 2–3 minutes. Turn and cook for 1–2 minutes longer for medium-rare, or until desired degree of doneness.

Place the tuna on a plate. Top with the poached egg and spoon on the salsa to serve.

Salmon, Avocado and Pistachio Wraps

Chopped pistachios add texture and flavor to these easily assembled wraps. Boston lettuce leaves may be substituted for the wraps according to taste.

SERVES 1

- ½ avocado, peeled, pitted and mashed
- ½ tsp. lime juice
- 3 Plantain Wraps (see recipe p. 160)
- 3 oz. cooked crumbled salmon
- 1 hard-cooked egg, peeled and coarsely chopped (see Chef's Tip)
- 1 tsp. chopped chives
- 2 tsps. chopped pistachios

Combine the avocado and lime juice and mash into a paste. Lay the wraps flat on a work surface. Divide the mixture in three and spread it onto the wraps. Divide the salmon between the wraps. Sprinkle on the egg, chives and pistachios. Season with freshly ground pepper and roll up to serve.

Chef's Tip: Hard-cooked eggs should never be boiled because boiling makes them prone to overcooking. To hard-cook eggs, place the eggs into a deep saucepan in a single layer and add cold water to cover by 1 inch. Bring the water to a boil over high heat. Remove the pan from the heat and cover it. Allow the eggs to remain in the covered pan for 12 minutes. Remove the eggs from the hot water and submerge them in an ice bath until they are chilled through, about 10 minutes. If using right away, peel the eggs under running water. Hard-cooked eggs in the shell can be refrigerated up to 1 week.

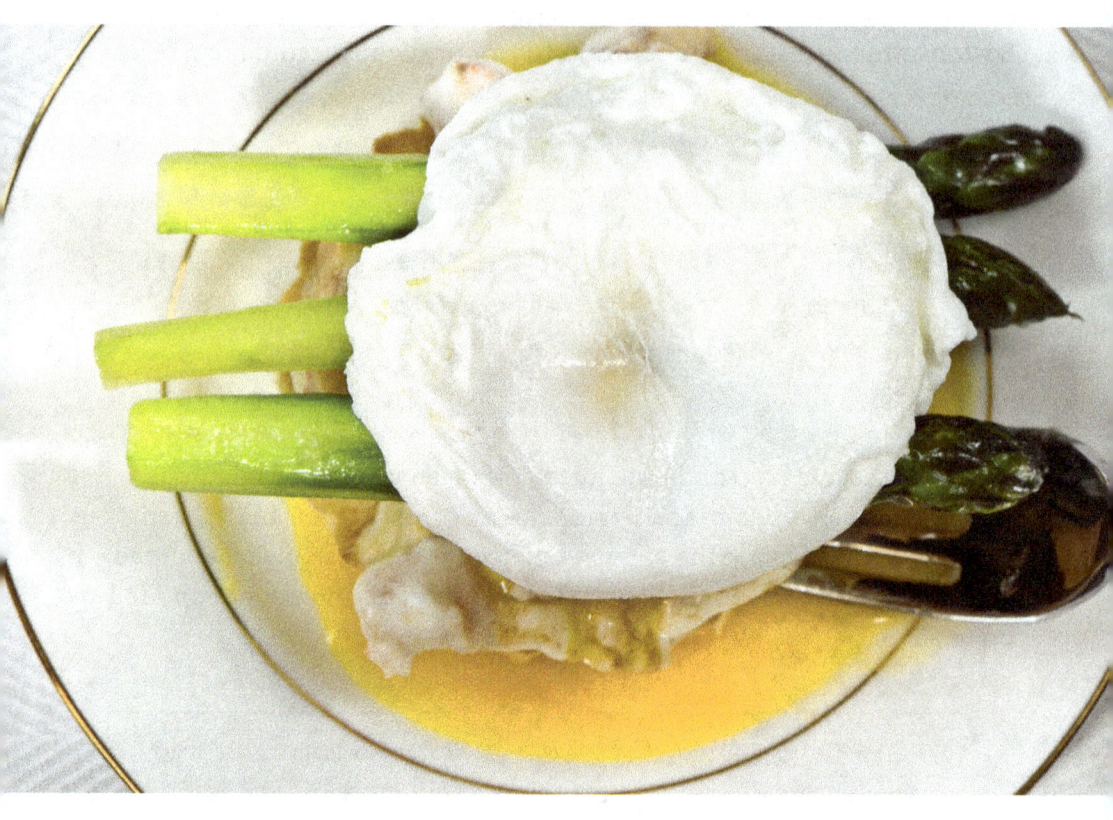

Eggs Lobster Oscar with Cauliflower

Eggs Lobster Oscar with Cauliflower

When you have time to enjoy a leisurely breakfast, try this tasty version of the classic eggs Oscar featuring sautéed lobster. Cauliflower provides the base for this eggs Benedict-style dish, topped with lobster, asparagus and a poached egg. Making a large lobster for the dinner recipe on p. 129 will yield extra meat for this dish.

SERVES 1

- 3 tsps. coconut oil
- 1 cup cauliflower florets, grated
- 1 tsp. chopped fresh tarragon (or substitute ¼ tsp. dried)
- 1 tsp. minced shallot
- 3–4 oz. cooked lobster meat, coarsely chopped
- 1 tbsp. coconut milk
- 3 asparagus peeled and blanched (see Chef's Tip below)
- 1–2 large eggs

Heat 1 tsp. coconut oil in a small skillet over medium heat. Add the cauliflower and cover. Cook for 4–5 minutes, stirring halfway through, until just softened. Remove from the heat and stir in the tarragon. Keep warm.

Heat 1 tsp. coconut oil in a small skillet over medium heat. Add the shallot and cook for 1–2 minutes, until softened. Add the lobster and coconut milk and cook for 1 minute, until milk is slightly thickened and lobster is heated through. Remove from the heat and keep warm.

Heat the remaining 1 tsp. oil in a small skillet over medium heat. Add the asparagus and sauté for 2–3 minutes, until heated through. Keep warm.

To poach the egg, fill a medium, deep skillet with about 2 ½" of water and bring the water to a boil. Lower the heat until the water is at a gentle simmer. Take a spoon and swirl it around the inner edge of the pan a few times to create a whirlpool effect. Immediately crack the egg and then hold it very close to the water to allow it to slip in gently. Slide a slotted spoon under the egg to keep it from sticking to the bottom and to collect the egg white into a ball around the yolk. (Add the second egg if serving and repeat the process.) Cover the pan and simmer the egg until the whites are set, 3–5 minutes depending on how runny you like the yolk. Remove the egg with a slotted spoon and blot it with a paper towel.

Mound the cauliflower in the center of the plate and press it into a ½-inch-thick circle. Spoon on the lobster. Set the asparagus on top of the lobster and set the poached egg on top to serve.

Chef's Tip: Blanching brightens and fixes the color of green vegetables and also allows them to retain a crisp texture when cooked. To blanch the asparagus (or other green vegetables), bring salted water to a boil in a medium skillet. Add the asparagus and cook for 2–3 minutes, until the asparagus turn green but are still crisp. Remove the asparagus and plunge them into an ice bath to stop the cooking. Allow to cool completely, then drain and blot dry with paper towels.

Hard-Cooked Eggs with Crab, Avocado and Belgian Endive

A delicious variation on traditional egg salad flavored with fresh dill and served on crisp Belgian endive leaves. The recipe may be assembled the night before, wrapped tightly in plastic wrap and stored in the refrigerator. Substitute Boston lettuce or Napa cabbage leaves if the endive is unavailable.

SERVES 1

- 2 tsps. mayonnaise (see recipe p. 163)
- 1 tbsp. chopped avocado
- ¼ tsp. lemon juice
- ¼ tsp. smoked paprika
- 2 hard-cooked eggs, shelled and coarsely chopped (see Chef's Tip p. 35)
- 3–4 oz. lump crabmeat
- 4 Belgian endive leaves
- 1 tsp. chopped dill

In a small bowl, combine the mayonnaise, avocado, lemon juice and smoked paprika until smooth. Fold in the eggs and crabmeat. Divide the mixture evenly among the endive leaves. Season with freshly ground black pepper and sprinkle on the chopped dill to serve.

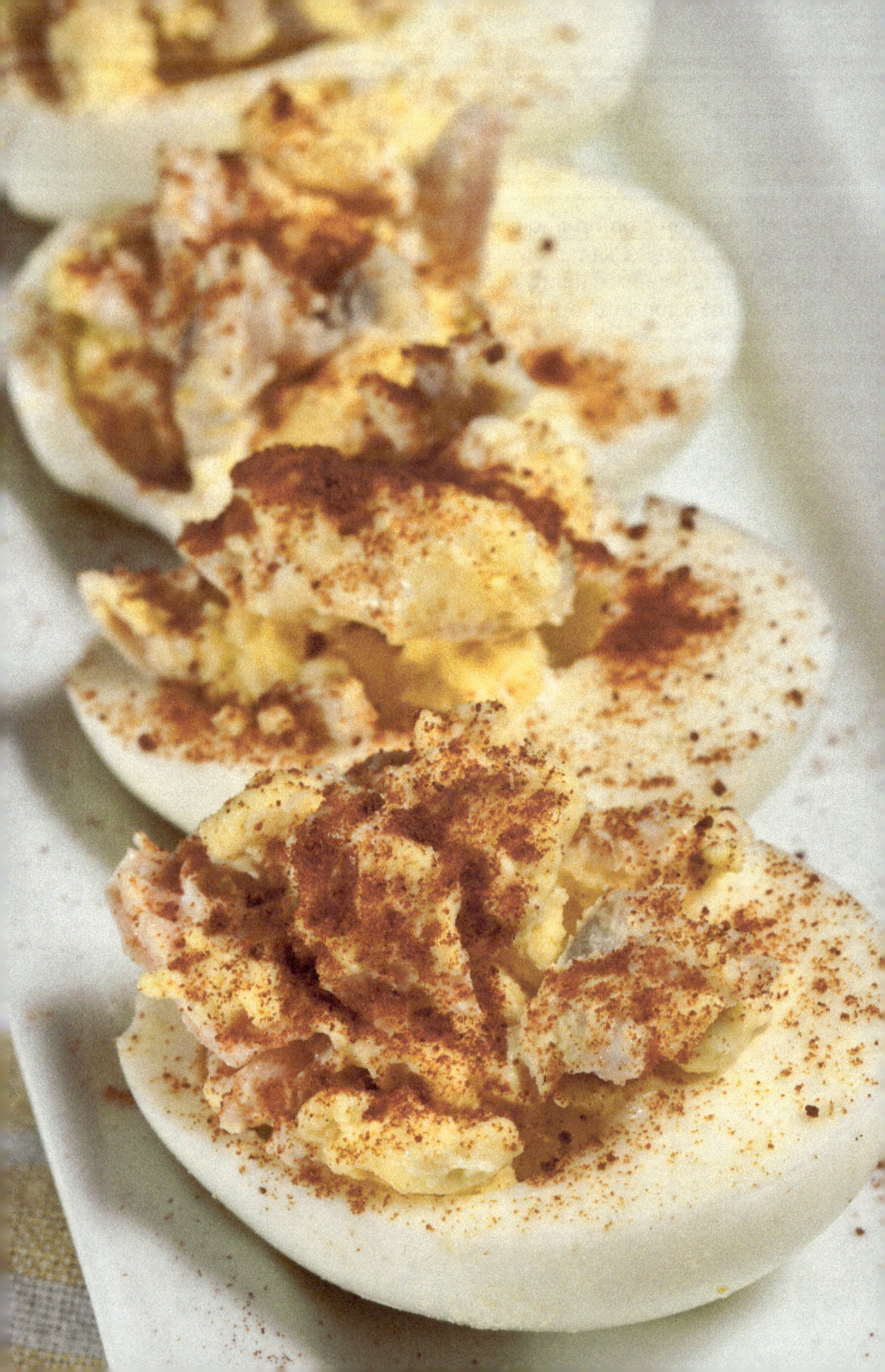

Salmon Deviled Eggs

A little effort turns ordinary deviled eggs into a special breakfast treat. Cooking some extra salmon at dinner on p. 139 will simplify the preparation.

SERVES 1

- 2 large hard-cooked eggs, cut in half lengthwise (see Chef's Tip p. 35)
- 2 tsps. mayonnaise (see recipe p. 163)
- ½ tsp. lemon juice
- 2 oz. cooked salmon filet, crumbled
- ¼ tsp. celery seeds
- 4 dill sprigs (optional)

Remove the yolks from the eggs and mash them in a small bowl. Add the mayonnaise and lemon juice and whisk to combine. Fold in the salmon and celery seeds and season with freshly ground pepper.

Divide the filling evenly among the egg white halves and place the dill sprigs if using on top to serve.

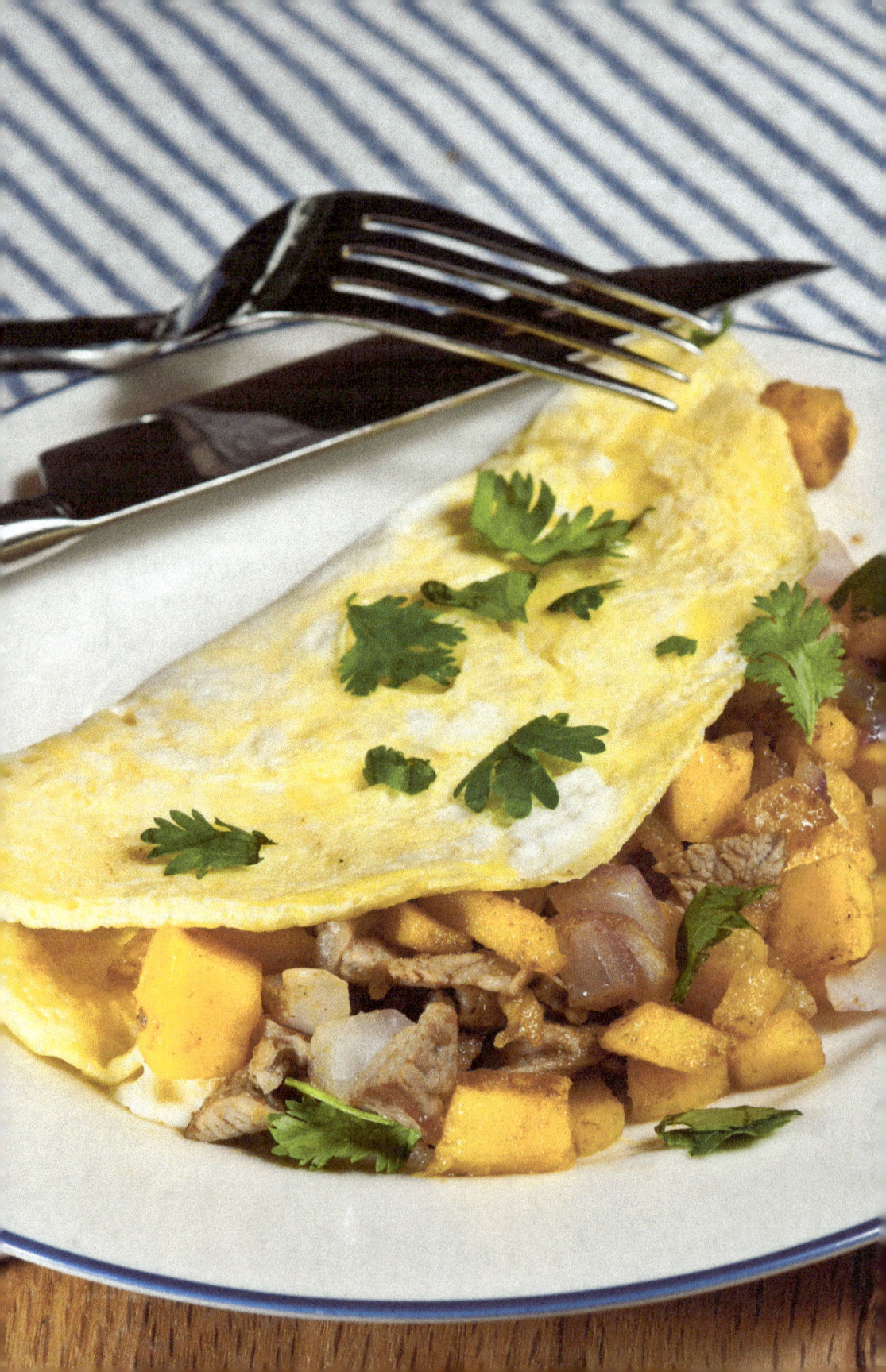

Pork and Mango Omelet

Fresh tropical flavor shines through in this easy-to-prepare omelet. The beaten egg is cooked in a thin, even layer, similar to a crepe, and then stuffed with the naturally sweet and savory filling. The combination of pork and mango gets an added kick from fresh jalapeno. Make extra pork tenderloin for the dinner on p. 145 to simplify the preparation.

SERVES 1

- 2 tsps. coconut oil
- 3 oz. cooked pork tenderloin, cut into ½" dice
- ¼ mango, peeled, seeded and cut into ½" dice
- ¼ jalapeno, peeled, seeded and minced
- ¼ tsp. finely grated ginger
- ¼ tsp. ground turmeric
- 1 tsp. lime juice
- 2 large eggs
- 1 tsp. chopped cilantro

Heat 1 tsp. coconut oil in a small skillet over medium heat. Add the pork, mango, jalapeno, ginger and turmeric, and stir until mango is softened and pork is just heated through, about 3-4 minutes. Remove from the heat. Stir in the lime juice and keep warm.

Whisk the eggs together in a small bowl and season with freshly ground pepper. Heat the remaining 1 tsp. oil in a small skillet over medium heat. Pour the eggs into the center of the pan and begin stirring them immediately for 30 seconds. Stop stirring, tilt the pan as necessary to cover the bottom with egg and allow the omelet to set up for 30 seconds. Carefully flip and cook on the other side until just cooked through, about 15-20 seconds longer. Remove from the heat.

Spoon the pork/mango mixture over half of the omelet. Run a spatula around the edge and fold the omelet in half. Place the omelet on a plate and sprinkle on the cilantro to serve.

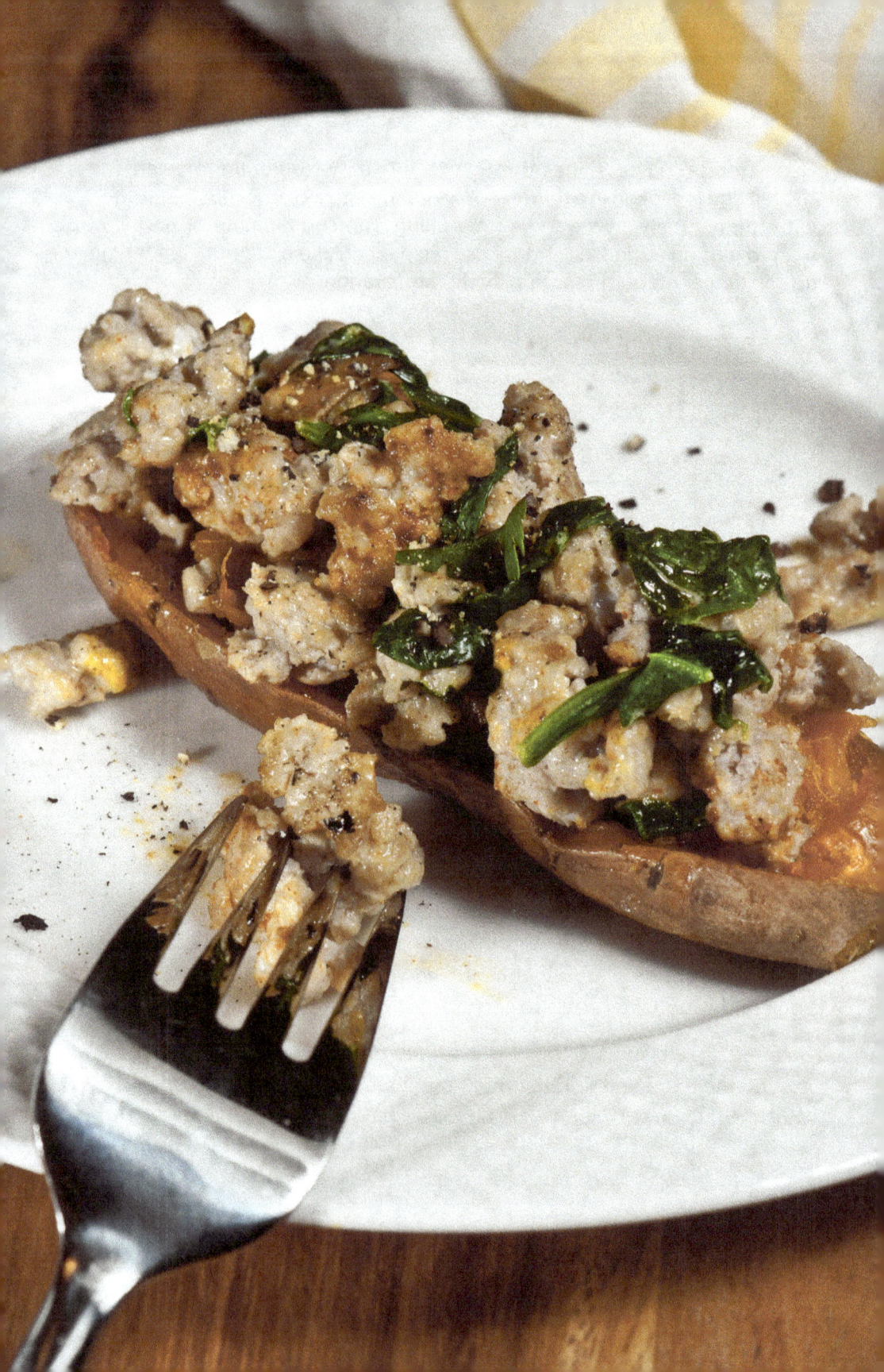

Sweet Potato Skin with Spinach and Italian Sausage

This satisfying breakfast dish is also delicious any time of the day. The crispy potato skin makes the perfect base for the savory sausage stuffing. To simplify the preparation, bake the sweet potato while you are roasting other items and refrigerate it until ready to use.

SERVES 1

- ½ baked sweet potato (see Chef's Tip)
- ¼ tsp. cayenne pepper
- 2 tsps. coconut oil
- ½ tsp. chopped shallot
- 3–4 oz. Italian sausage (see recipe p. 176)
- 1 cup baby spinach
- 1 tbsp. coconut milk
- 1 tsp. pine nuts (optional)

Preheat the oven to 375 degrees F. Lightly grease a baking sheet.

Scrape the sweet potato out of the peel into a small bowl. Add the cayenne pepper and mash to combine.

Lightly brush the sweet potato skin with 1 tsp. coconut oil and set on the baking sheet. Bake for 5–7 minutes, until skin is crisp.

In the meantime, heat the remaining 1 tsp. oil in a small skillet over medium heat. Add the chopped shallot and Italian sausage and sauté until sausage is just cooked through, about 4–5 minutes. Add the spinach and cook until just wilted, about 1 minute. Stir in the coconut milk and remove from the heat. Season with freshly ground black pepper.

Remove the skin from the oven and fill it with the mashed sweet potato. Spoon on the sausage and spinach mixture. Bake for 4–5 minutes, until top is lightly browned and the potato is heated through. Sprinkle on the pine nuts if using to serve.

Chef's Tip: To bake a sweet potato, preheat the oven to 400 degrees F and line a baking sheet with foil. Wash and dry the potato and pierce it several times all over with a fork. For a dry, crispy skin (if you are simply eating the potato), brush the outside with a little coconut oil and bake uncovered for 45–60 minutes until tender. For a softer skin (for use in the recipe above), wrap each sweet potato in foil and bake for 45–60 minutes until tender.

Portobello, Sausage and Egg Stack

Layers of sausage and eggs between two portobello caps make a delicious, satisfying breakfast. Broiling or grilling the mushrooms the night before and reheating them briefly would save a little time in the morning. While it is not necessary to remove the gills from portobello mushrooms, they will discolor the dish and make it less appealing visually.

SERVES 1

- 3 tsps. extra virgin olive oil
- 2 medium portobello mushroom caps, gills removed
- 2 oz. Italian sausage, pressed into a 3–4" patty (see recipe p. 176)
- 1 large egg

Heat 2 tsps. olive oil in a medium skillet over medium heat. Season the mushroom caps with pepper and add them to the pan, gill side up. Cook the mushrooms until they begin to sweat, about 3-4 minutes. Turn the mushrooms over and cook on the other side until tender and cooked through, about 2-3 minutes longer. Remove from the pan, placing one cap gill side up on a plate.

In the meantime, heat the remaining 1 tsp. of oil in a small skillet over medium heat. Add the sausage patty to the pan and cook for 3-4 minutes, until lightly browned. Turn the sausage and cook for 2-3 minutes longer, until just cooked through. Place the sausage on top of the portobello cap. Add the egg to the skillet and cook for 1 minute until the outer edges begin to set. Add 1 tbsp. water to the pan, place the lid on and lower the heat. Cook for 2-3 minutes longer until the yolk is set and egg white is opaque. Place the cooked egg on top of the sausage and cover with the second portobello to serve.

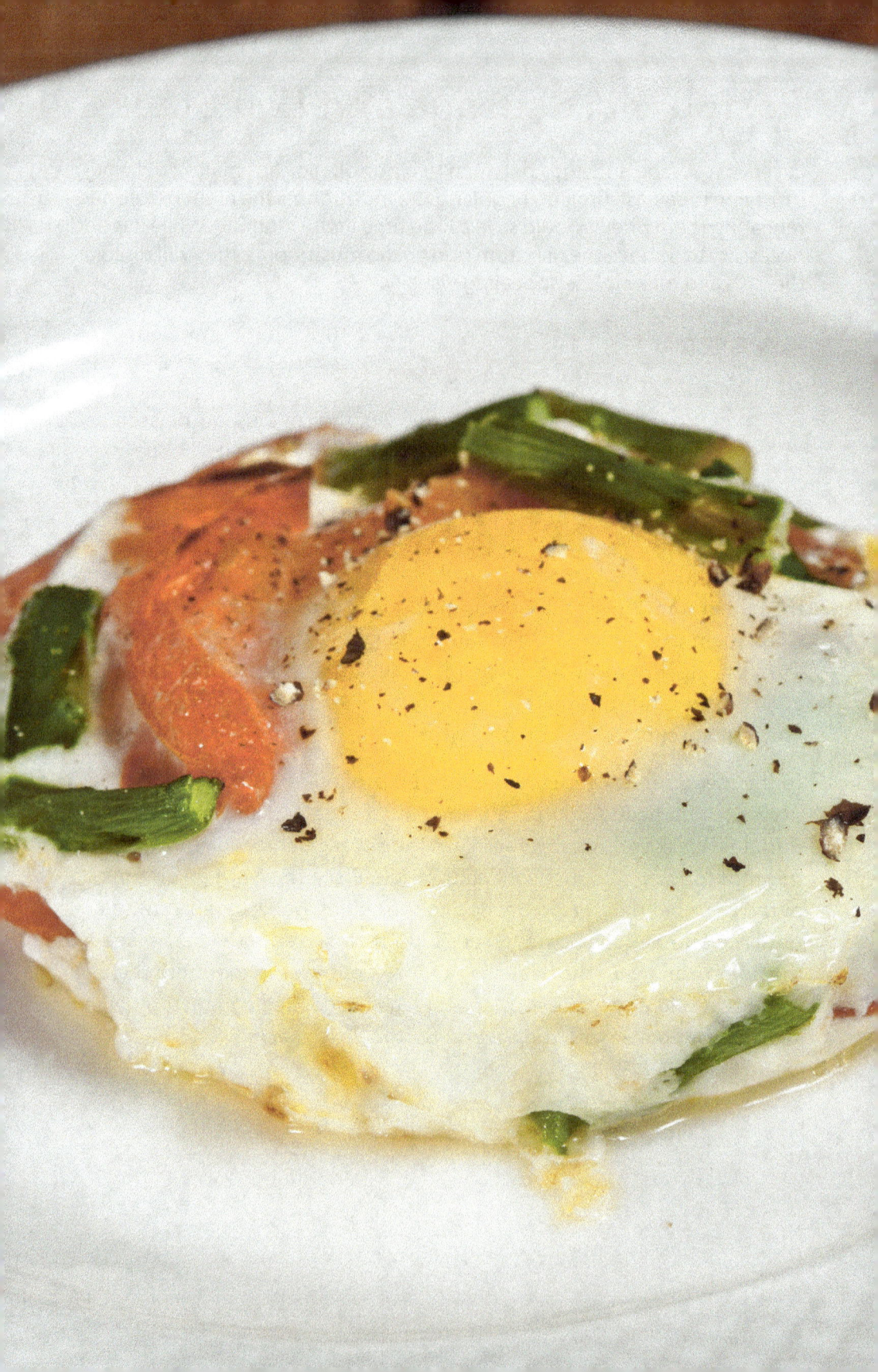

Asparagus, Egg and Tomato Tart

In this version of a tart, sliced tomato replaces the traditional crust. Lining the baking dish with parchment will make it easier to unmold the baked egg tart.

SERVES 1

- 1 plum tomato, cut into ¼" thick slices
- ¼ tsp. dried oregano
- 4 spears asparagus, blanched and cut into 1" pieces
- 1 tsp. extra virgin olive oil
- 1 large egg

Preheat the oven to 425 degrees F. Line an individual tart pan or small baking dish with parchment and lightly grease the parchment.

Layer the tomatoes in the bottom of the dish and sprinkle on the oregano. Bake for 10 minutes. Layer the blanched asparagus on top of the tomato. Drizzle on the olive oil and season with freshly ground pepper. Cook for 4–5 minutes, until asparagus are lightly browned and softened. Crack the egg on top of the asparagus. Bake for 8–10 minutes longer, until the white is just set but the yolk is still runny.

Drain off any excess liquid from the tomato and allow the dish to cool slightly. Carefully remove the parchment and season with freshly ground pepper to serve.

Italian Fried Eggs with Sausage and Peppers

Olive oil imparts a unique flavor to these over-medium eggs, served over a sauté of sweet peppers and Italian sausage. Italian frying peppers are long and conical, with a slightly sweet, mild flavor—but substitute bell pepper if unavailable.

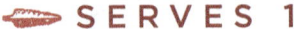 **SERVES 1**

- 2 tsps. extra virgin olive oil
- ½ green Italian frying pepper, trimmed, seeded and cut into ⅛" strips
- 2 oz. crumbled Italian sausage (see recipe p. 176)
- 2 large eggs

Heat 1 tsp. olive oil in small skillet over medium. Add the pepper and cook for 4–5 minutes, until softened and edges are lightly browned. Add the sausage and cook for 3–4 minutes, until just cooked through. Remove from the heat and spoon the mixture onto a plate. Cover and keep warm.

Wipe out the skillet and heat the remaining 1 tsp. olive oil over medium heat. Crack the eggs into the skillet and lower the heat. Cook until the whites become opaque, about 2 minutes. Turn the eggs and cook for 1 minute longer. Immediately remove the eggs from the pan and place them onto the sausage pepper mixture. Season with freshly ground pepper to serve.

Pumpkin, Pecan and Coconut Breakfast Bowl

Eating eggs for breakfast every day can seem repetitious, no matter how well they are prepared. Breakfast bowls and soups are a tasty way to bring variety to the morning meal while still staying with the plan. Shredded pumpkin adds texture to this savory breakfast dish. Add a few ounces of chopped or shredded pork for a more robust meal.

SERVES 1

- 1 tbsp. coconut oil
- 1 cup fresh shredded pumpkin (see Chef's Tip)
- ¼ tsp. freshly grated nutmeg
- ¼ tsp. ground cinnamon
- ½ cup vegetable or chicken stock
- 2 tbsps. coconut milk
- ¼ tsp. vanilla extract
- 1 tsp. chopped pecans
- 1 tbsp. large unsweetened toasted coconut flakes

In a small saucepan, melt the coconut oil over medium-high heat. Add the fresh pumpkin and sauté for 2–3 minutes. Stir in the nutmeg and cinnamon. Add the stock and bring to a boil. Lower heat to a simmer, cover and cook until the pumpkin is tender, about 10–12 minutes.

Drain off any excess liquid. Stir in the coconut milk and vanilla. Cook for 1 minute and remove from the heat. Sprinkle on the chopped pecans and toasted coconut flakes to serve.

Chef's Tip: For shredded pumpkin, select a smaller "pie" pumpkin, about 1–2 lbs. Cut a wide circle around the stem through the flesh and remove and discard the top piece. Scoop out the insides and reserve seeds for toasting if desired. Cut the pumpkin into quarters. Cut each quarter into half again. Remove the skin with a knife or vegetable peeler. Use a box grater or food processor to shred the pumpkin.

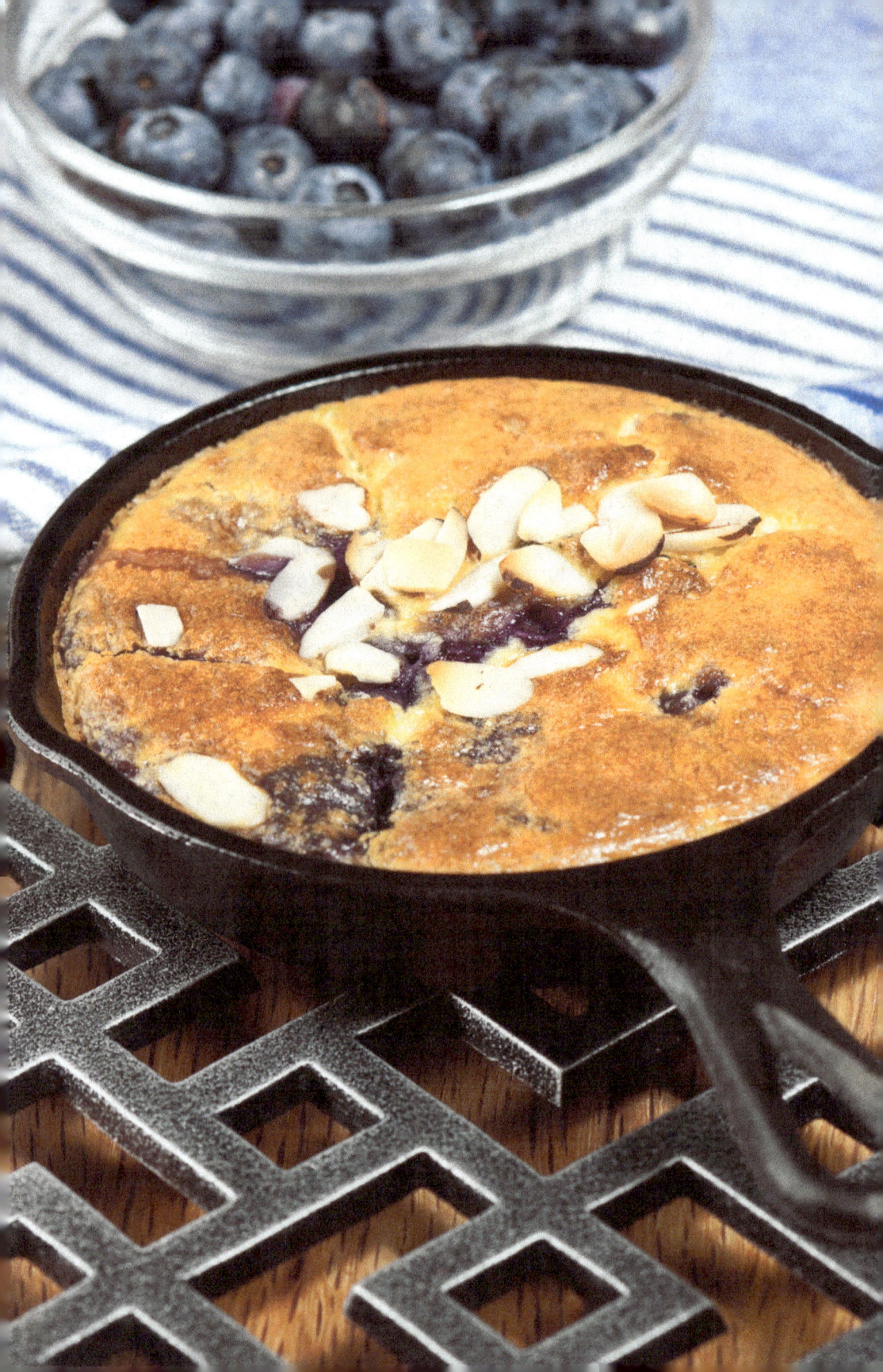

Blueberry Almond Custard

True to its origins in French cuisine without the addition of sugar, this clafoutis-style custard is flavored with chopped apple and ripe blueberries for a satisfying breakfast dish. If fresh local berries are out of season, substitute frozen wild blueberries from Maine if available.

SERVES 1

- ¼ apple, peeled, seeded and coarsely chopped
- 2 tbsps. coconut milk
- 1 large egg
- ½ tsp. vanilla extract
- 2 tbsps. almond flour or meal
- ½ cup blueberries
- 1 tsp. sliced almonds

Preheat oven to 375 degrees F. Grease an individual cast-iron skillet or tart pan.

In a food processor, combine the apple, coconut milk, egg and extract and process until smooth. Add the almond flour and process until smooth.

Place the blueberries in the prepared pan. Pour the batter over the blueberries. Sprinkle sliced almonds over batter.

Bake until golden and set, about 35–40 minutes. Serve warm or cool.

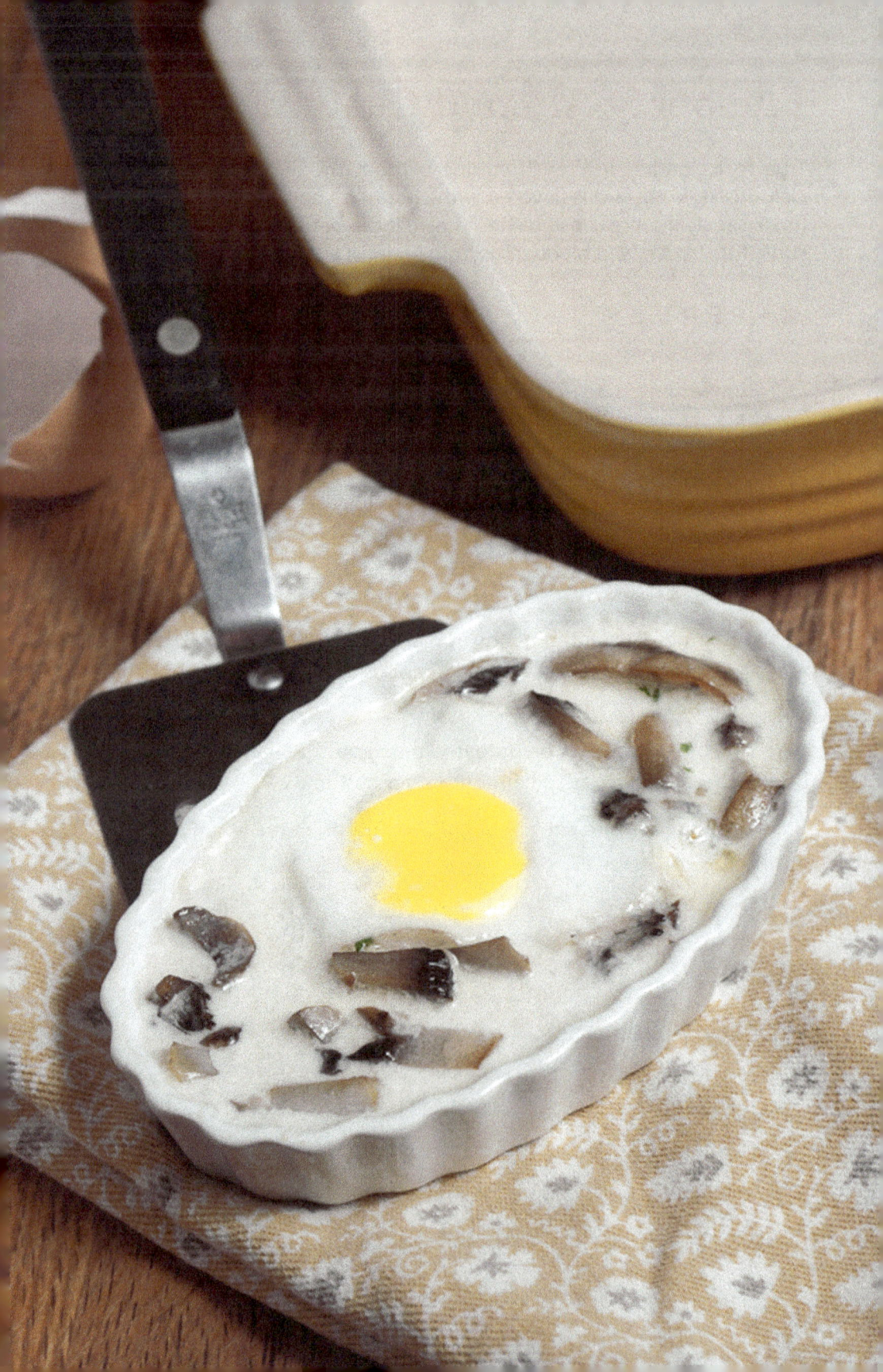

Coddled Egg with Sun-Dried Tomatoes and Mushrooms

Coddling is a gentle self-steaming method that produces tender cooked whites and a runny yolk, similar to a soft-cooked egg. The amount of time to cook the egg will vary according to the type of baking dish you use (less for a wider, shallower ramekin) and according to how runny you like the yolk. Sauté 1 oz. ground pork or turkey with the mushrooms for a more substantial dish.

SERVES 1

- 1 tsp. extra virgin olive oil
- ¼ tsp. minced shallot
- ¼ cup chopped mushrooms
- 1 sun-dried tomato, soaked in water and thinly sliced
- 1 large egg

Heat the olive oil in a small skillet. Add the shallot, mushrooms and sun-dried tomato and sauté until softened, about 4–5 minutes. Remove from the heat and set aside.

Place an individual ramekin into a large skillet or saucepan (with a lid) and add cold water until the water level is about halfway up the side of the dish. Remove the ramekin and bring the water to a boil over high heat. Lower the heat to a simmer.

Lightly grease the ramekin and spoon the mushroom mixture into it. Crack the egg into the ramekin. Place the lid onto the pan. Cook the egg for 4–7 minutes, until the whites are set and the yolks are cooked according to the desired degree of doneness. Season the egg with freshly ground pepper to serve.

Baked Tomato with Caramelized Onions and Egg

This baked tomato is filled with sweet onions and topped with creamy soft-scrambled eggs. Add ground turkey or pork to the stuffing for a more substantial dish.

SERVES 1

- ¼ cup caramelized onions (see Chef's Tip)
- 1 medium slicing tomato, cored
- 1 tsp. extra virgin olive oil
- 1 tsp. chopped fresh thyme
- ¼ tsp. crushed red pepper
- 1 tsp. pine nuts
- 1 large egg, lightly beaten
- 1 tsp. chopped flat-leaf parsley

Preheat the oven to 450 degrees F. Line a baking sheet with foil.

Spoon the onions into the tomato and place it on the baking sheet. Bake for 12–15 minutes, until the tomato is softened. Sprinkle on the thyme, red pepper and pine nuts.

Whisk the egg in a small bowl or measuring cup. Heat the olive oil in a small skillet over medium heat. Pour the egg into the skillet and cook, stirring constantly, for 3–4 minutes, until curds are formed but eggs are still wet. Remove from the heat and continue stirring until eggs are glossy. Spoon the egg into the tomato. Sprinkle on the parsley and season with freshly ground pepper to serve.

Chef's Tip: To caramelize the onions, heat 1 tsp. coconut or olive oil in a small skillet over medium-high heat. Add 1 cup of sliced onion and stir to coat. Lower the heat and cook until softened and golden, stirring occasionally, about 35–40 minutes.

Swiss Chard, Pork Belly and Bell Pepper Frittata

Super green Swiss chard pairs with sweet bell pepper in this simple –to-prepare Italian omelet. Pork belly differs from bacon in that it is cooked without the addition of cures and preservatives. The recipe requires preparing it ahead of time (it may also be purchased cooked, but check the ingredients for added salt), so it is optional but worth the extra effort.

SERVES 1

- 1 tbsp. extra virgin olive oil
- 2 tbsps. chopped onion
- ½ tsp. minced garlic
- 1 cup coarsely chopped Swiss chard, stems removed
- ¼ red or yellow bell pepper, seeded and chopped
- ½ tsp. lemon juice
- 2 oz. cooked pork belly, optional (see recipe p. 177)
- 2 large eggs
- 1 tsp. chopped chives

Preheat the broiler to high and set the rack 3-4 inches from the heat.

Heat the olive oil in a small ovenproof skillet over medium-high heat. Add the onion and cook until softened, about 4-5 minutes. Add the garlic and sauté for 30 seconds. Add the Swiss chard and pepper. Lower the heat and cook until the vegetables are tender, about 4-5 minutes. Stir in the lemon juice and pork belly if using.

Whisk together the eggs in a small bowl until frothy. Add the eggs to the Swiss chard mixture and stir for 2-3 minutes, until the eggs begin to set. Continue cooking without stirring for 2-3 minutes longer, until the eggs are set on the bottom but the top is still moist.

Place the frittata under the broiler and cook for 2-3 minutes longer, until lightly browned and cooked through. Sprinkle on the chives and season with freshly ground pepper to serve.

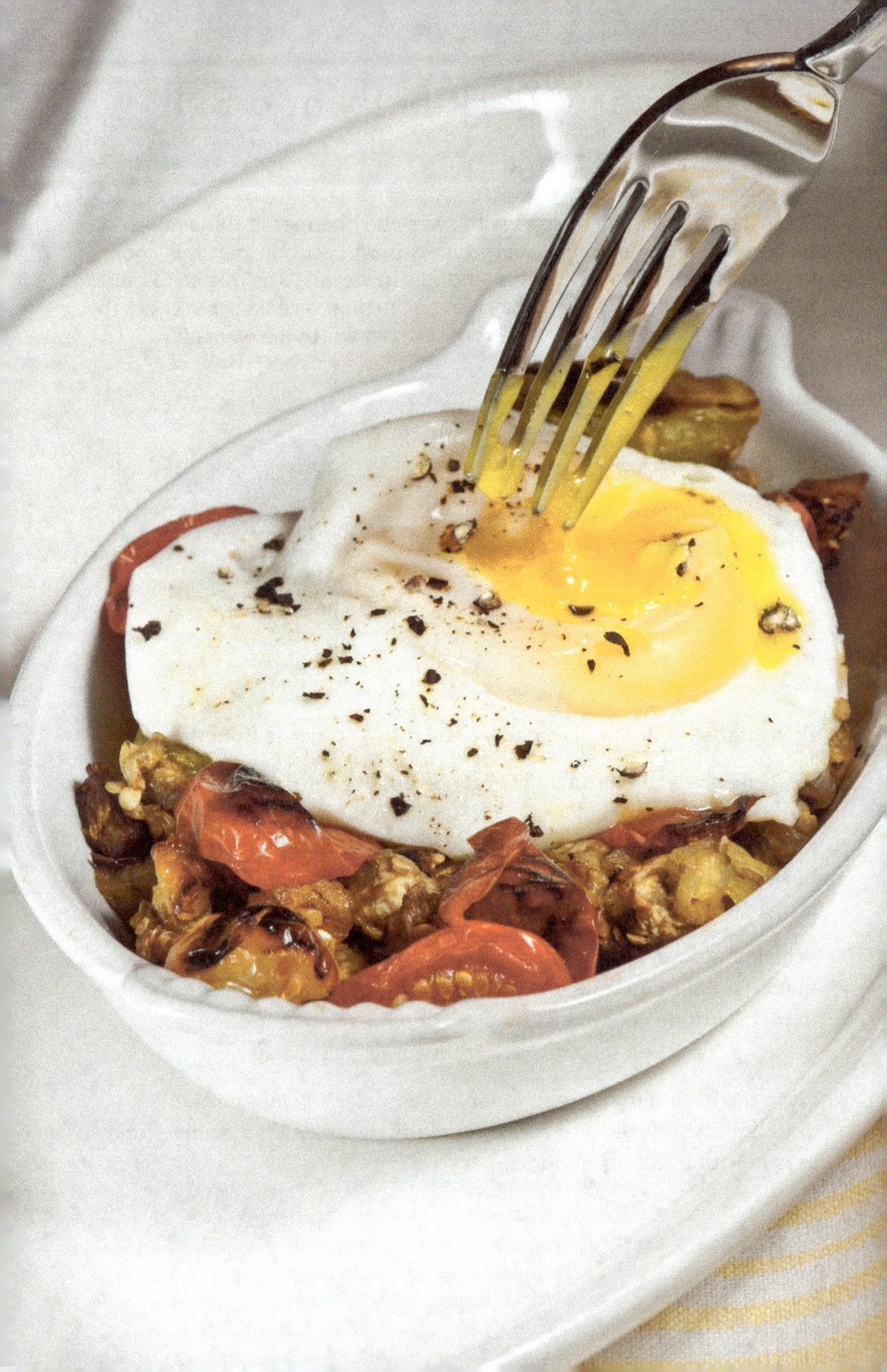

Roasted Eggplant and Cherry Tomatoes with Egg

Roasting the eggplant adds flavor to this tasty breakfast, topped with a sunny-side up egg.

SERVES 1

- ¼ medium eggplant, peeled and diced (about ½ cup)
- 1 tbsp. chopped onion
- ½ tsp. crushed red pepper
- 2 tsps. extra virgin olive oil
- 6 cherry tomatoes, coarsely chopped
- 2 basil leaves, cut into chiffonade
- 1 large egg

Preheat oven to 400 degrees F. Lightly grease an individual cast-iron skillet or small baking dish.

Combine the eggplant, onion and crushed red pepper in the skillet. Drizzle on 1 tsp. olive oil. Bake the eggplant for 20–25 minutes, until just tender. Add the tomatoes and stir to combine. Bake for 5–7 minutes longer, until tomatoes are just softened. Season with freshly ground black pepper and sprinkle on the basil.

In the meantime, prepare the egg sunny-side up. In a small non-stick skillet, heat the remaining 1 tsp. olive oil over medium heat. Crack the egg into the pan (alternatively, crack it into a small bowl and slide it into the pan). Cook for 1 minute until the outer edges begin to set. Add 1 tbsp. water to the pan, place the lid on and lower the heat. Cook for 2–3 minutes longer until yolk is set and egg white is opaque. Place the egg on top of the eggplant and tomatoes to serve.

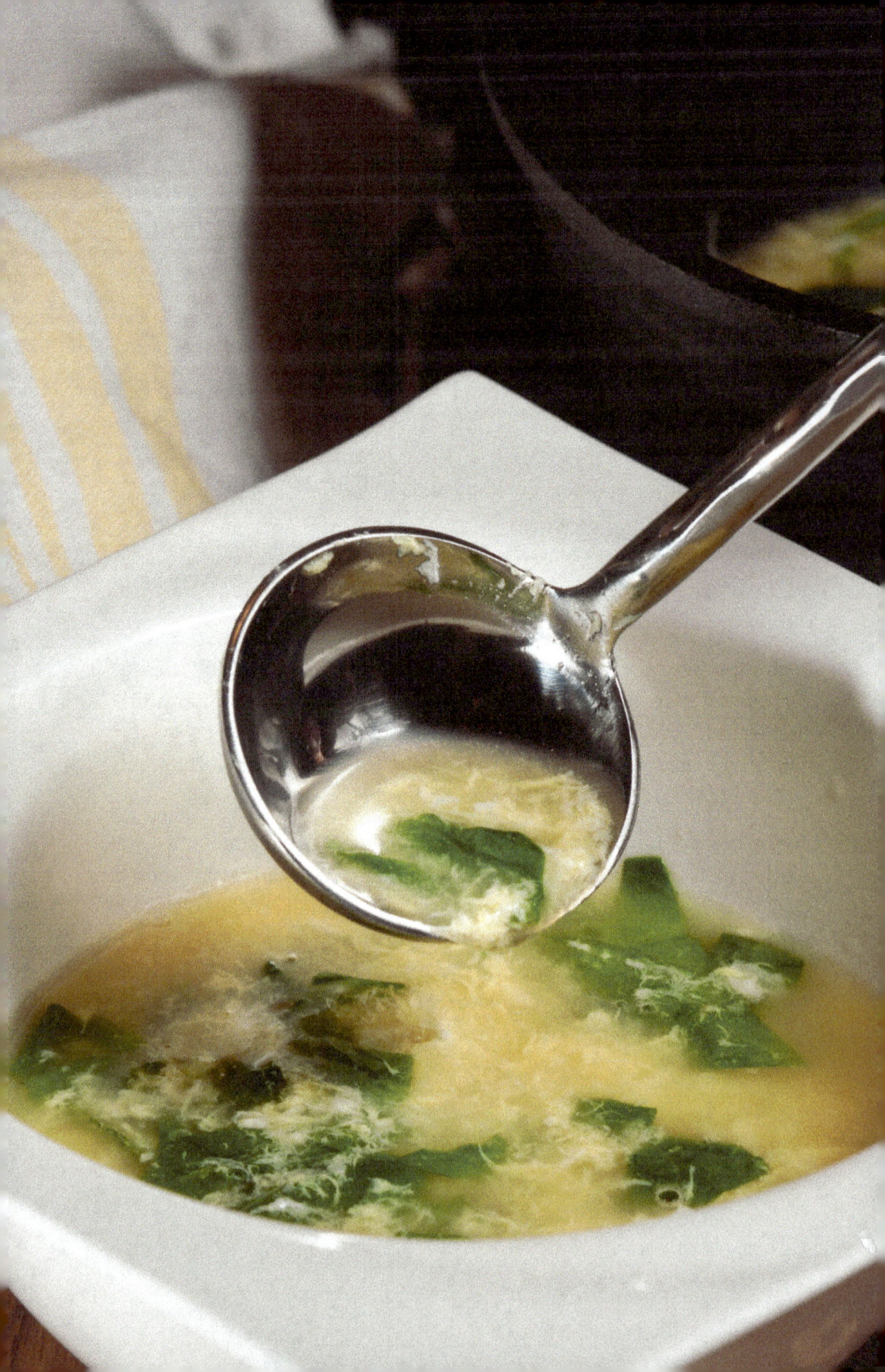

Scrambled Egg Soup with Spinach

This comfort food breakfast is inspired by an Italian soup known in Italy as stracciatella (which translates as "little shred"). Here, spinach replaces the traditional Parmesan cheese. Add shredded chicken for a more substantial meal.

SERVES 1

- 1 cup chicken stock
- ½ tsp. crushed red pepper
- 2 large eggs, lightly beaten
- 1 cup baby spinach, cut into chiffonade
- 1 tsp. lemon juice
- 1 tsp. chopped flat-leaf parsley

Combine the stock and crushed red pepper in a medium saucepan over medium-high heat. Bring to a boil, then lower the heat to a simmer and whisk the eggs into the stock. Add the spinach and cook until just wilted, about 30 seconds. Remove from the heat and season with freshly ground pepper. Stir in the lemon juice and sprinkle on the parsley to serve.

Bok Choy, Carrot and Radish Omelet Soup

This Thai-inspired soup incorporates eggs as part of the dish, but the vegetables definitely take center stage. Add shredded chicken or pork for a more substantial meal. Commercial chili powder often includes salt and sugar, so check the label and make your own if necessary (see recipe p. 162).

SERVES 1

- 1 large egg
- 1 scallion, trimmed and coarsely chopped
- 1 tsp. chopped cilantro
- 1 tsp. coconut oil
- 1 ½ cups vegetable or chicken stock
- ½ tsp. chili powder
- ½ tsp. turmeric
- 1 medium carrot, finely diced
- 1 radish, trimmed and finely diced
- 1 baby bok choy, trimmed and shredded
- 1 tsp. lime juice

Whisk the egg in a small bowl until frothy. Stir in the scallion and cilantro. Heat the oil in a small skillet over medium heat. Add the egg mixture and swirl the pan to evenly distribute the egg. Cook until the omelet is cooked on the bottom but still glossy on the top, about 2 minutes (this will help it stick together when it is rolled). Remove the omelet from the pan and immediately roll it up. Allow the omelet to rest for 2-3 minutes. Thinly slice the omelet into rings and set aside.

Combine the stock, chili powder and turmeric in a medium saucepan. Bring to a boil over medium-high heat. Add the carrot, radish and bok choy and simmer until the vegetables are tender but still slightly crisp, about 3-4 minutes. Add the omelet pieces and cook for 1 minute longer. Pour the mixture into a bowl and stir in the lime juice to serve.

Five Spice Chicken and Egg Scramble

The flavor of five spice powder paired with ginger and scallion adds an Asian-inspired twist to traditional scrambled eggs. Freezing fresh ginger makes it easy to grate finely and preserves the flavor.

SERVES 1

- 1 tsp. coconut oil
- ½ tsp. finely grated ginger
- ½ tsp. five spice powder
- 3 shitake mushrooms, stems removed and thinly sliced
- 3 oz. shredded cooked chicken (see Chef's Tip)
- 1 scallion, trimmed and coarsely chopped
- 2 large eggs, lightly beaten

Heat the coconut oil in a small skillet over medium heat. Add the ginger, five spice powder and mushrooms and stir until mushrooms are softened, about 4–5 minutes. Add the chicken and scallion and cook for 1 minute. Add the eggs to the pan and cook, stirring constantly, about 3–4 minutes, until curds are formed but eggs are still wet. Remove from the heat and continue stirring until eggs are glossy and just cooked. Season with freshly ground pepper to serve.

Chef's Tip: To poach a boneless, skinless chicken breast (6–8 oz.), place the chicken breast, 1 clove garlic and 4 peppercorns in a medium saucepan and add water to cover. Bring to a boil over medium-high heat. Cover the pan and reduce the heat to a simmer. Cook for 10–12 minutes, until just cooked through (internal temperature of 165 degrees F). Remove the chicken breast and allow it to cool before refrigerating. This poaching technique also works for turkey cutlets.

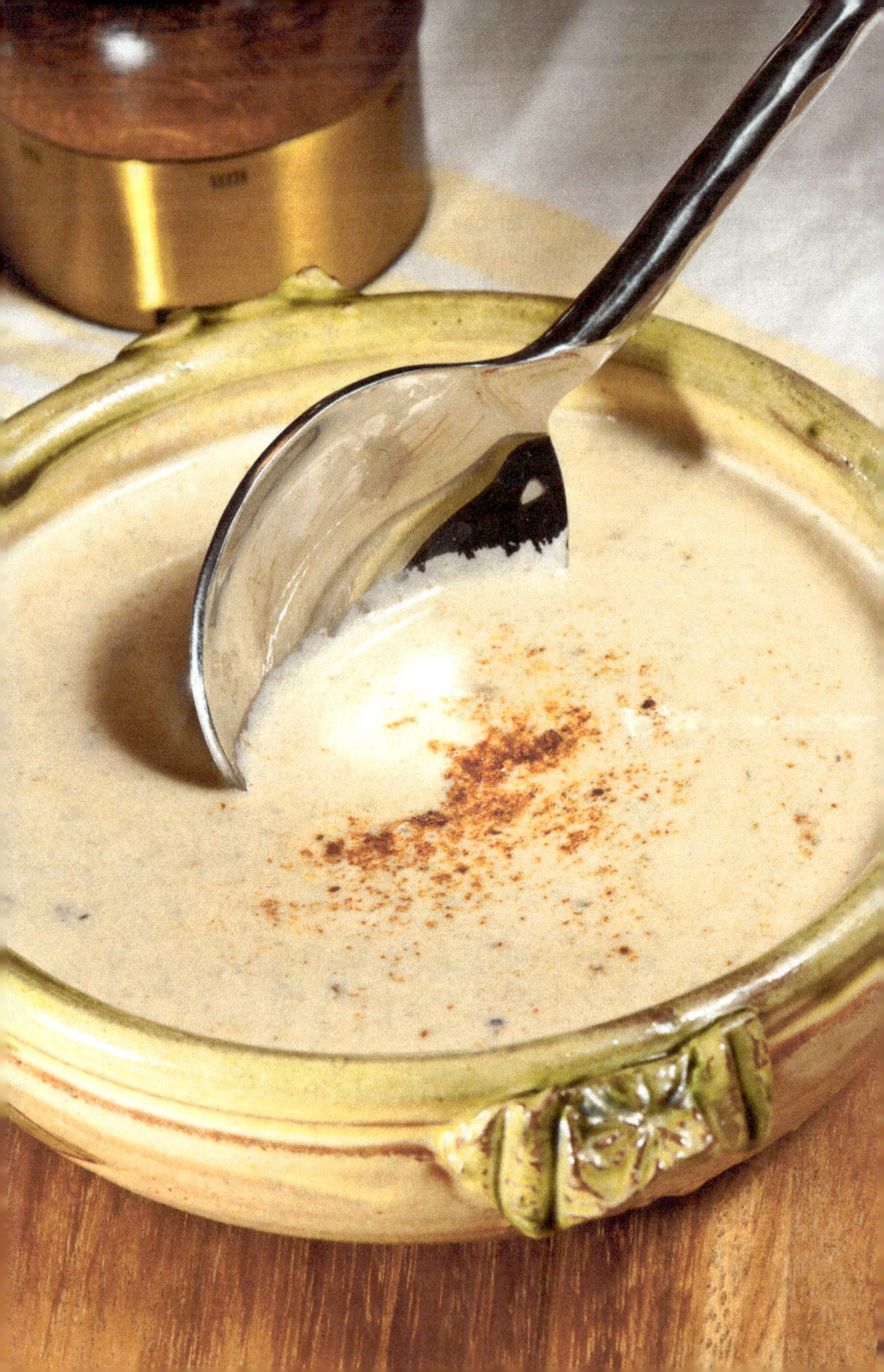

Turkey, Cauliflower and Apple Soup

Savory cauliflower and turkey combine in this hearty breakfast soup that is delicious any time of day.

SERVES 1

- 1 tsp. extra virgin olive oil
- 4 oz. ground turkey
- 1 ½ cups cauliflower florets (about ¼ large head)
- ½ apple, peeled, seeded and coarsely chopped
- 1 ½ cups chicken stock
- ¼ tsp. dried sage
- ½ tsp. cinnamon
- ¼ tsp. cayenne pepper

Heat the oil in a small skillet over medium heat. Add the turkey and sauté until cooked through, about 3–4 minutes. Remove the turkey and drain on paper towels. Set aside.

Combine the cauliflower, apple, stock, sage, cinnamon and cayenne pepper in a medium saucepan. Bring the mixture to a boil over medium-high heat, then reduce the heat to a simmer. Cook until cauliflower is tender, about 18–20 minutes.

Puree the mixture with a blender (or use an immersion blender) until smooth. Return the puree to the saucepan and bring to a boil over medium-high heat. Stir in the ground turkey and cook until heated through to serve.

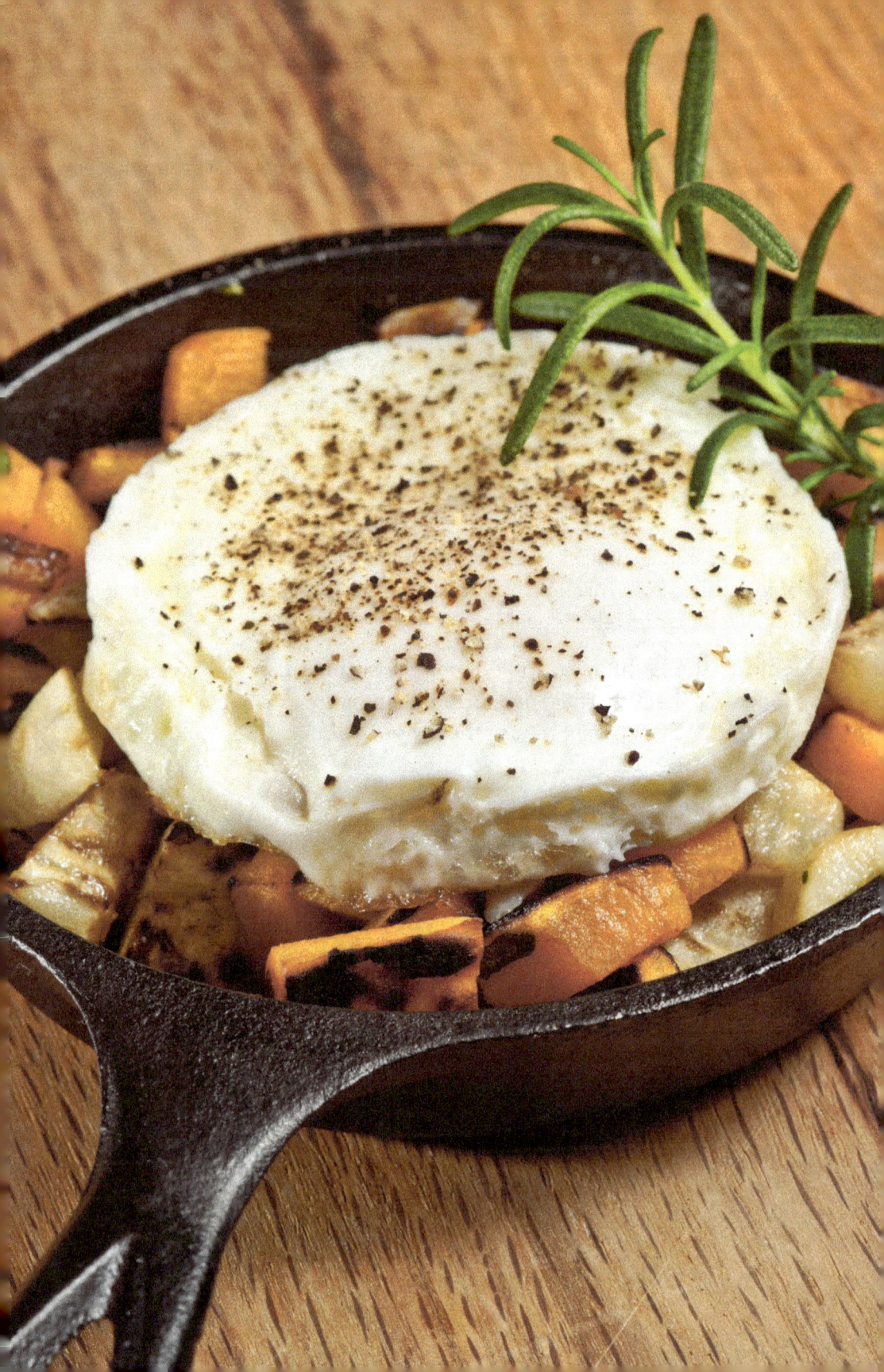

Sweet Potato Hash with Turkey and Egg

Chili powder and cayenne pepper add layers of flavor to this savory sweet potato hash, served with a sunny-side up egg in the center.

SERVES 1

- ¼ large sweet potato, peeled and cut into ½" dice
- ½ medium turnip, peeled and cut into ½" dice
- 3 tsps. extra virgin olive or coconut oil
- 2 tbsps. chopped sweet onion
- ½ tsp. chili powder
- ¼ tsp. cayenne pepper
- 1 tsp. chopped fresh rosemary
- 2 oz. cooked turkey, diced
- 1 large egg

Fill a medium, deep skillet with water and bring to a boil over medium-high heat. Add the sweet potato and turnip and cook until just tender, about 8–10 minutes. Drain off the water and dry the vegetables with paper towels.

Heat 2 tsps. oil in a small skillet over medium heat. Add the onion, sweet potato, turnip, chili powder and cayenne pepper and stir to combine. Cook, stirring occasionally, until the onion is softened and the vegetables are lightly browned, about 4–5 minutes. Stir in the rosemary and turkey and cook until the turkey is heated through, about 1 minute longer. Set aside and keep warm.

Heat the remaining 1 tsp. oil in a small skillet over medium heat. Crack the egg into the pan (alternatively, crack it into a small bowl and slide it into the pan). Cook for 1 minute until the outer edges begin to set. Add 1 tbsp. water to the pan, place the lid on and lower the heat. Cook for 2–3 minutes longer until yolk is set and egg white is opaque. Set the egg on top of the hash and season with freshly ground pepper to serve.

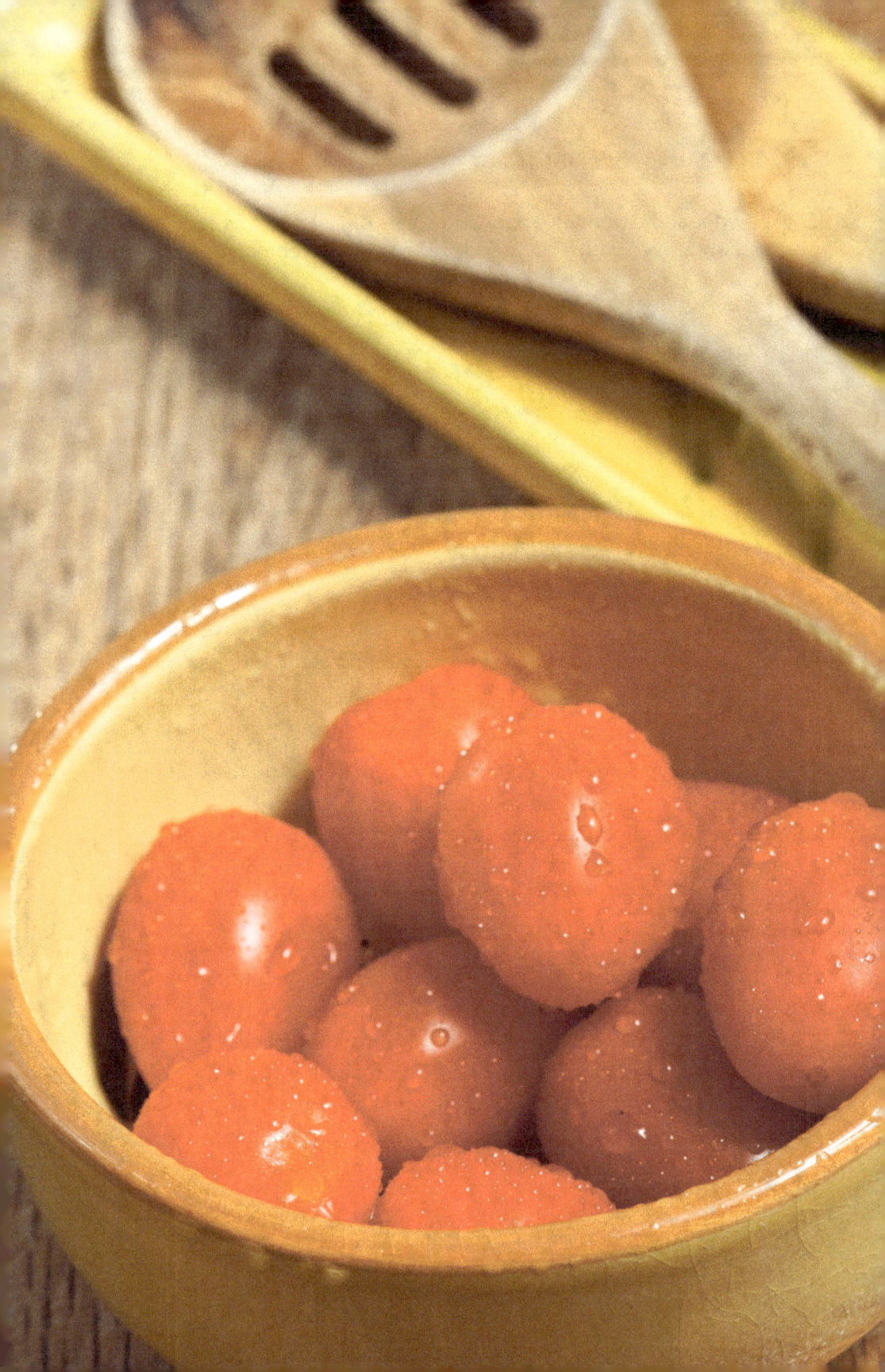

CHAPTER TWO
25 Lunches

- Veal Scallops with Cherry Tomatoes and Celery
- Steak with Mango, Arugula and Pistachios
- Beef Short-Rib and Vegetable Soup
- Tuna Filet with Saffron Slaw
- Seafood and Butternut Squash Chowder
- Chilled Cucumber, Avocado and Shrimp Soup
- Seafood and Avocado Salad
- Crab, Fennel and Asparagus Salad
- Shrimp, Red Pepper and Almond Soup
- Shrimp Papaya Salad with Cashews
- Roasted Beets with Salmon, Walnuts and Mint
- Pork Tenderloin with Spinach, Orange and Onions
- Watermelon, Cucumber and Red Onion with Pork
- Celery Root, Leek and Pork Belly Soup
- Cabbage, Carrot and Apple Slaw with Chicken
- Chicken Salad with Carrot, Radish and Cucumber
- Spaghetti Squash Primavera with Chicken
- Spicy Chicken Salad with Mustard Greens
- Turkey with Roasted Sweet Potato, Turnip and Pear
- Chicken and Coconut Soup with Cauliflower

- Watercress and Sweet Potato Soup
- Curried Zucchini Spinach Soup
- Roasted Eggplant and Tomato Soup
- Wild Mushroom Soup
- Spicy Sweet Potato and Parsnip Soup

Veal Scallops with Cherry Tomatoes and Celery

Veal cutlets are lightly pounded, quickly pan-fried with lemon and garlic and finished with a refreshing salad of cherry tomatoes and celery.

SERVES 1

- 1 ½ tbsps. extra virgin olive oil
- 2 tsps. lemon juice
- ½ tsp. lemon zest
- 1 tsp. chopped flat-leaf parsley
- ¼ tsp. chopped sage
- ½ tsp. crushed red pepper
- 8 cherry tomatoes, halved
- 2 celery stalks, trimmed and sliced on the diagonal into ½" pieces
- 2 (2 oz.) veal cutlets, pounded out to ⅛"
- ½ tsp. minced garlic

Combine 1 tbsp. olive oil, 1 tsp. lemon juice, lemon zest, parsley, sage and crushed red pepper in a small bowl. Add the cherry tomatoes and celery and toss to combine. Set aside.

Season the veal with freshly ground pepper. Heat the remaining ½ tbsp. olive oil in a medium skillet over medium heat. Add the garlic and cook for 30 seconds. Add the veal and sauté for 1 minute. Turn and cook for 1 minute longer, until no longer pink. Remove from the heat and sprinkle on the remaining 1 tsp. lemon juice (the veal may be refrigerated if not serving immediately).

Place the veal on a plate and spoon on the tomato/celery mixture to serve.

Steak with Mango, Arugula and Pistachios

This quick-to-prepare steak dredged in pistachios is delicious served warm or cool. The mango salsa adds a tropical flair.

SERVES 1

- 4 oz. sirloin or other tender steak
- ¼ tsp. smoked paprika
- 1 ½ tsps. finely ground pistachios
- 2 tsps. coconut oil
- 1 tbsp. extra virgin olive oil
- 1 tsp. lime juice
- ½ tsp. chopped thyme
- 1 cup arugula
- 1 scallion, trimmed and coarsely chopped
- ½ mango, peeled, seeded and coarsely chopped
- 1 tsp. toasted large coconut flakes

Season the steak with freshly ground pepper. Combine the paprika and 1 tsp. pistachios in a small bowl. Lightly brush the steak with ½ tsp. coconut oil and dredge the steak in the pistachios to coat.

Heat the remaining 1 tsp. coconut oil in a small skillet over medium-high heat. Add the steak and sear until lightly browned, about 2 minutes. Turn the steak and cook 1 ½–2 minutes longer for medium rare, or according to desired degree of doneness. Remove from the pan and allow the steak to rest for at least 5 minutes.

Whisk the olive oil, lime juice, thyme and remaining 1 tsp. pistachios in a medium bowl. Add the arugula, scallion, mango and coconut flakes and toss to coat. Thinly slice the steak and layer it over the salad to serve.

Beef Short-Rib and Vegetable Soup

The ribs in this rich vegetable soup simmer for a few hours but are well worth the wait. The soup freezes well, so it makes sense to make extra and enjoy it on several occasions. You may also want to cook extra short-ribs and reserve the meat to add to salads, wraps and other soups. Refrigerating the soup before serving helps congeal any excess fat, making it easier to skim off.

SERVES 1

- 1 tbsp. olive oil
- 3 tbsps. chopped onion
- ½ lb. beef short-ribs
- 1 garlic clove, peeled and crushed
- 3 plum tomatoes, peeled, seeded and diced
- 1 ½ cups beef stock
- ½ tsp. freshly ground pepper
- ½ tsp. dried thyme
- ¼ tsp. dried oregano
- 1 bay leaf
- 1 tsp. orange zest
- ¼ cup sliced okra
- 1 carrot, peeled and diced
- 1 celery stalk, trimmed and diced
- 1 cup beet greens, rinsed well, stemmed and cut into ½" ribbons
- 2 tsps. chopped flat-leaf parsley

In a large saucepan or cast-iron Dutch oven, heat the oil over medium-high heat. Add the onion and cook until softened, about 4–5 minutes. Add the short-ribs, garlic and tomatoes and stir to coat. Add the beef stock, ½ cup water, pepper, thyme, oregano, bay leaf and orange zest. Bring to a boil over medium-high heat. Cover and reduce the heat to a simmer. Cook for 2–2 ½ hours, until the meat is very tender. Use a slotted spoon to remove the meat and bones from the pot into a bowl. Allow the meat to cool slightly, and discard the bones. Trim off any remaining fat and shred the beef into large chunks.

Strain the broth and any juices from the meat through a fine mesh sieve set over a bowl and discard the solids. Skim off any fat that rises to the surface. Return the liquid to the pot and bring to a boil over medium-high heat. Add the okra and simmer for 10 minutes. Add the carrot, celery and reserved beef to the soup and simmer for 5 minutes. Add the beet greens and simmer for 5–7 minutes longer, until vegetables are just tender. Stir in the parsley to serve.

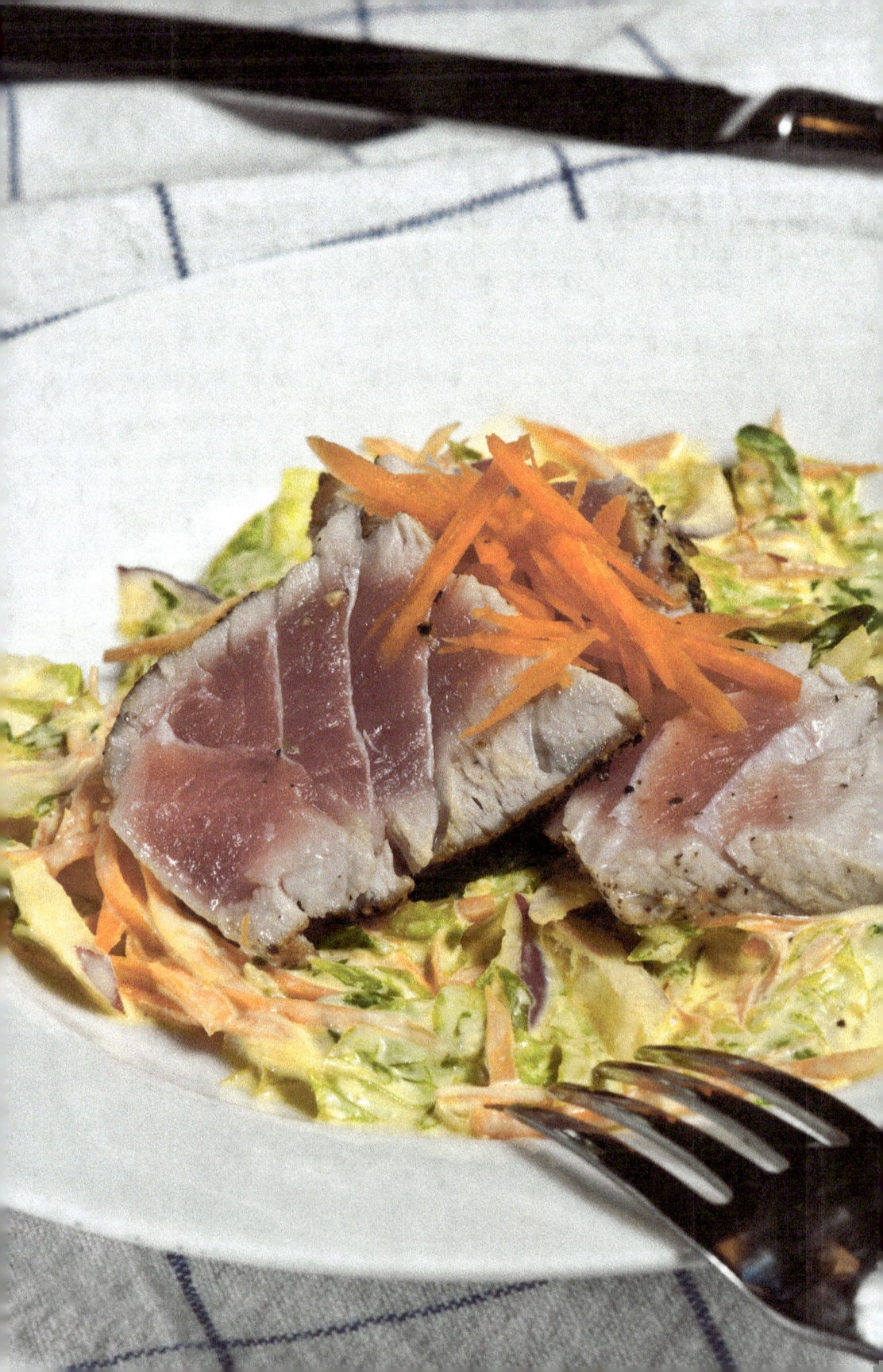

Tuna Filet with Saffron Slaw

Fresh tuna cooks in minutes and is paired with a creamy vegetable slaw. Pan-sear an extra piece of tuna ahead of time when making the dinner on p. 133 or see the Chef's Tip if you need to cook it closer to serving.

SERVES 1

- Pinch saffron threads
- 1 tbsp. mayonnaise (see recipe p. 163)
- ¼ tsp. minced garlic
- 1 tsp. lemon juice
- Pinch dry mustard
- ½ cup shredded Napa cabbage
- ½ medium carrot, peeled and julienned
- 1 radish, trimmed and julienned
- 1 tsp. chopped cilantro
- 3–4 slices pan-seared tuna steak (about 4 oz.), cut into 1" pieces (see Chef's Tip)

Soak the saffron in 2 tsps. warm water in a small bowl for 10 minutes. Whisk together the mayonnaise, garlic and lemon juice in a medium bowl. Add the mustard and saffron with water and whisk to combine.

Add the cabbage, carrot and radish to the dressing and toss to coat. Season with freshly ground pepper and sprinkle on the cilantro. Top with the tuna slices to serve.

Chef's Tip: To pan-sear the tuna, season a 4 oz. tuna steak with freshly ground pepper. Heat 1 tsp. olive oil in a small skillet over medium-high heat. Sear the tuna for 2 minutes, then turn and sear the other side for 1–2 minutes longer for medium-rare or until desired degree of doneness.

Seafood and Butternut Squash Chowder

Vegetables pureed with coconut milk add a slightly creamy texture to this delicious variation of the classic seafood soup.

SERVES 1

- ½ cup butternut squash cubes (about ¼ butternut squash)
- 1 carrot, peeled and diced
- 2 tsps. extra virgin olive oil
- 3 tbsps. chopped sweet onion
- 1 tsp. minced shallot
- ½ tsp. finely grated ginger
- ½ cup cauliflower florets
- ¼ tsp. dried thyme
- ¼ cup coconut milk
- 1 ½ cups fish or chicken stock
- 1 bay leaf
- 4 oz. skinless halibut or other white flaky fish, cut into chunks
- 7–8 large (31–35 per lb.) shrimp, peeled, deveined and halved
- ¼ lb. small clams, scrubbed, steamed and removed from the shell (see Chef's Tip)
- 1 tsp. chopped chives

Slice 3 of the butternut squash cubes into ½" dice and reserve in a small bowl. Add half of the diced carrot to the bowl and set aside.

Heat the olive oil in a medium saucepan or cast-iron Dutch oven over medium heat. Add the onion, remaining ½ carrot, shallot and ginger and cook until the onion is softened, about 4-5 minutes. Add the remaining squash cubes, cauliflower and thyme and stir for 1 minute. Add the coconut milk, stock and bay leaf and bring to a boil. Lower to a simmer and cook until the squash is tender, about 25-30 minutes.

Remove the bay leaf and puree the mixture in a blender (or use an immersion blender) until smooth. Bring the chowder to a simmer over medium heat in a medium saucepan. Add the remaining squash and carrots and cook for 5 minutes. Add the halibut and cook for 2 minutes. Add the shrimp and cook until they turn pink, about 2-3 minutes.

Add the clams and remove from the heat. Season with freshly ground black pepper and garnish with chives to serve.

Chef's Tip: To steam the clams, bring 1 cup of water to a boil in a medium saucepan. Add the clams and cover the pot. Steam the clams until they just open, about 12–15 minutes. Remove the opened clams from the pan and discard any unopened ones.

To puree hot liquids with a blender, remove the small cap from the blender lid (the pour lid) and cover the lid with a kitchen towel. The steam from the hot soup will be able escape without forcing the blender lid to pop off.

Fill the blender no more than halfway with soup. Start the blender on low to allow steam to escape and gradually increase the speed. Repeat as necessary until all is pureed.

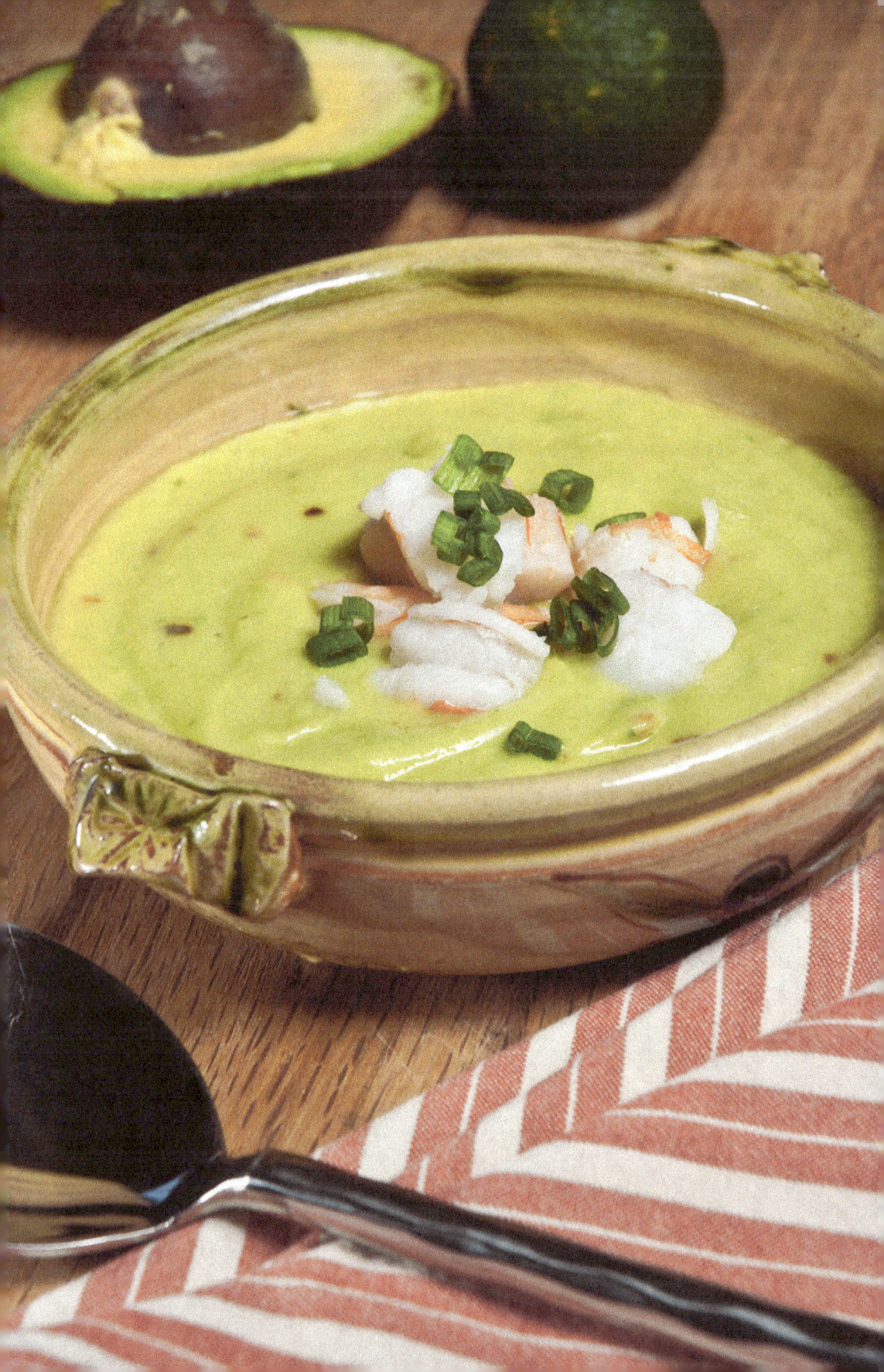

Chilled Cucumber, Avocado and Shrimp Soup

This refreshing chilled soup is delicious any time of the day, especially in warmer weather.

SERVES 1

- 1 medium cucumber, peeled
- ½ avocado, pitted and peeled
- 1 scallion, trimmed and coarsely chopped
- 1 tbsp. lime juice
- 2 tsps. chopped dill
- ¼ tsp. crushed red pepper
- ¼ tsp. celery seed
- ¼ tsp. paprika
- 7–8 large (31–35 per lb.) cooked shrimp, coarsely chopped

In a food processor or blender, combine the cucumber, avocado, scallion, lime juice, dill, red pepper, celery seed, paprika and half the shrimp with ¼ cup cold water. Process until smooth. Season with freshly ground pepper to taste and garnish with the remaining shrimp to serve.

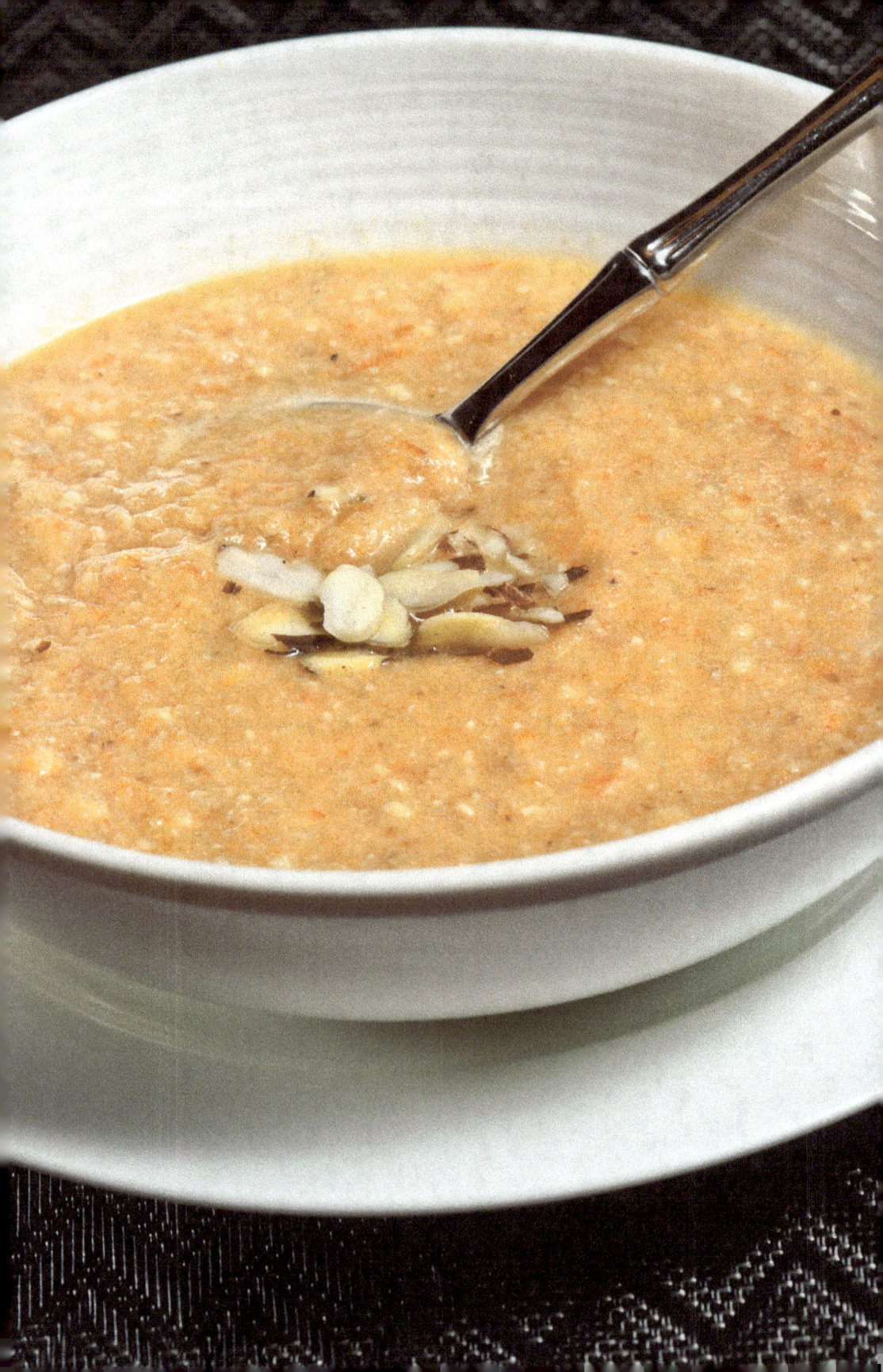

Shrimp, Red Pepper and Almond Soup

This hearty soup was inspired by Spanish romesco, a nut and roasted red pepper sauce. Ground almonds add a creamy texture and rich flavor to this blend of roasted pepper, tomatoes and shrimp.

SERVES 1

- 1 tbsp. extra virgin olive oil
- 3 plum tomatoes, peeled, seeded and coarsely chopped
- 1 tbsp. chopped onion
- 1 clove garlic
- 2 tbsps. chopped roasted red pepper (see Chef's Tip)
- ½ tsp. smoked paprika
- 1 ½ cups seafood, chicken or vegetable stock
- 7–8 large (31–35 per lb.) cooked shrimp, peeled and deveined
- 10 almonds, finely ground
- 1 tsp. lime juice
- 1 tsp. sliced almonds

Heat the olive oil in a medium saucepan over medium heat. Add the tomatoes, onion and garlic and lower the heat. Cook, stirring often, until the vegetables are slightly caramelized, about 10-12 minutes. Stir in the roasted pepper, smoked paprika and stock. Bring the mixture to a boil, then lower to a simmer. Cook for 18-20 minutes, until tomatoes are broken down.

Add the shrimp and cook for 2-3 minutes, until just cooked through and pink. Remove the mixture from the heat and allow to cool slightly. Stir in the almonds. Puree the mixture with a blender (or use an immersion blender) until almost smooth. Stir in the lime juice, sprinkle on the sliced almonds and season with freshly ground pepper to serve.

Chef's Tip: How to Roast Bell Peppers

Method One: On a gas stovetop, place the pepper directly in the flame and turn it, using heatproof tongs, until the skins are charred. Alternatively, if you have an electric stovetop, place the pepper directly under the broiler and proceed as above.

Method Two: This method makes sense if you are already using the oven to prepare other food. Preheat the oven to 400 degrees F. Place the peppers on a rimmed baking sheet and roast for 1 hour, turning occasionally for even browning.

To peel the roasted peppers, immediately seal them in foil (alternatively, place them in a paper bag) and allow them to steam to loosen the skin. Rub the peppers with paper towels to remove the skin and rinse under running water.

Seafood and Avocado Salad

The basis for this tasty salad is a seafood-enhanced guacamole that also makes an excellent dip. Crisp romaine adds texture to the dish.

SERVES 1

- ½ avocado, pitted and peeled
- 1 tsp. chopped fresh cilantro
- 1 tsp. chopped onion
- 1 tsp. minced jalapeno
- 1 tsp. lime juice
- 1 tsp. orange juice
- 2 oz. fresh crabmeat
- 7–8 large (31–35 per lb.) cooked shrimp, peeled, deveined and coarsely chopped
- 3 oz. cooked lobster (optional)
- 1 cup romaine lettuce, cut into ½" pieces

Mash the avocado in a medium bowl or with a mortar and pestle. Add the cilantro, onion, jalapeno, lime juice and orange juice and stir to combine. Fold in the crabmeat, shrimp and lobster (if using). Fold in the lettuce and season with freshly ground pepper to serve.

Crab, Fennel and Asparagus Salad

Crisp fennel is delicious raw, and adds a light anise accent to this salad, balanced by the natural sweetness of the crab. Use a mandolin if available to slice the fennel into thin, even slices.

SERVES 1

- 1 tbsp. avocado or olive oil
- 1 tsp. lemon juice
- 1 tsp. chopped fresh mint
- ¼ tsp. celery seed
- ½ medium fennel bulb, cored and thinly sliced (about 1 cup)
- ½ pear, seeded and thinly sliced
- 4 asparagus spears, blanched and sliced in half lengthwise
- 4 oz. crabmeat
- 2 tsps. chopped pecans

Combine the oil, lemon juice, mint and celery seed in a medium bowl. Add the fennel, pear, asparagus and crab and toss to coat. Season with freshly ground pepper and sprinkle on the pecans to serve.

Shrimp Papaya Salad with Cashews

This refreshing Vietnamese-style salad features shrimp paired with crisp vegetables and fresh mint.

SERVES 1

- ¼ green papaya (or ½ medium jicama), peeled and julienned (about 1 cup)
- 1 medium carrot, peeled and julienned
- 1 tbsp. avocado oil
- 1 tsp. crushed red pepper
- 1 Thai chili, seeded and minced
- ¼ tsp. minced garlic
- 3 tbsps. chopped fresh mint
- 7–8 large (31–35 per lb.) cooked shrimp, tails removed, sliced in half lengthwise
- 1 tbsp. fresh lime juice
- 2 tbsps. chopped cashews

Spread papaya and carrot on paper towels and roll up to squeeze out as much liquid as possible. In a large bowl, whisk together the avocado oil, red pepper, chili, garlic and mint. Add the papaya and carrot and toss to coat. Add the shrimp and lime juice and toss to combine. Sprinkle on the chopped cashews to serve.

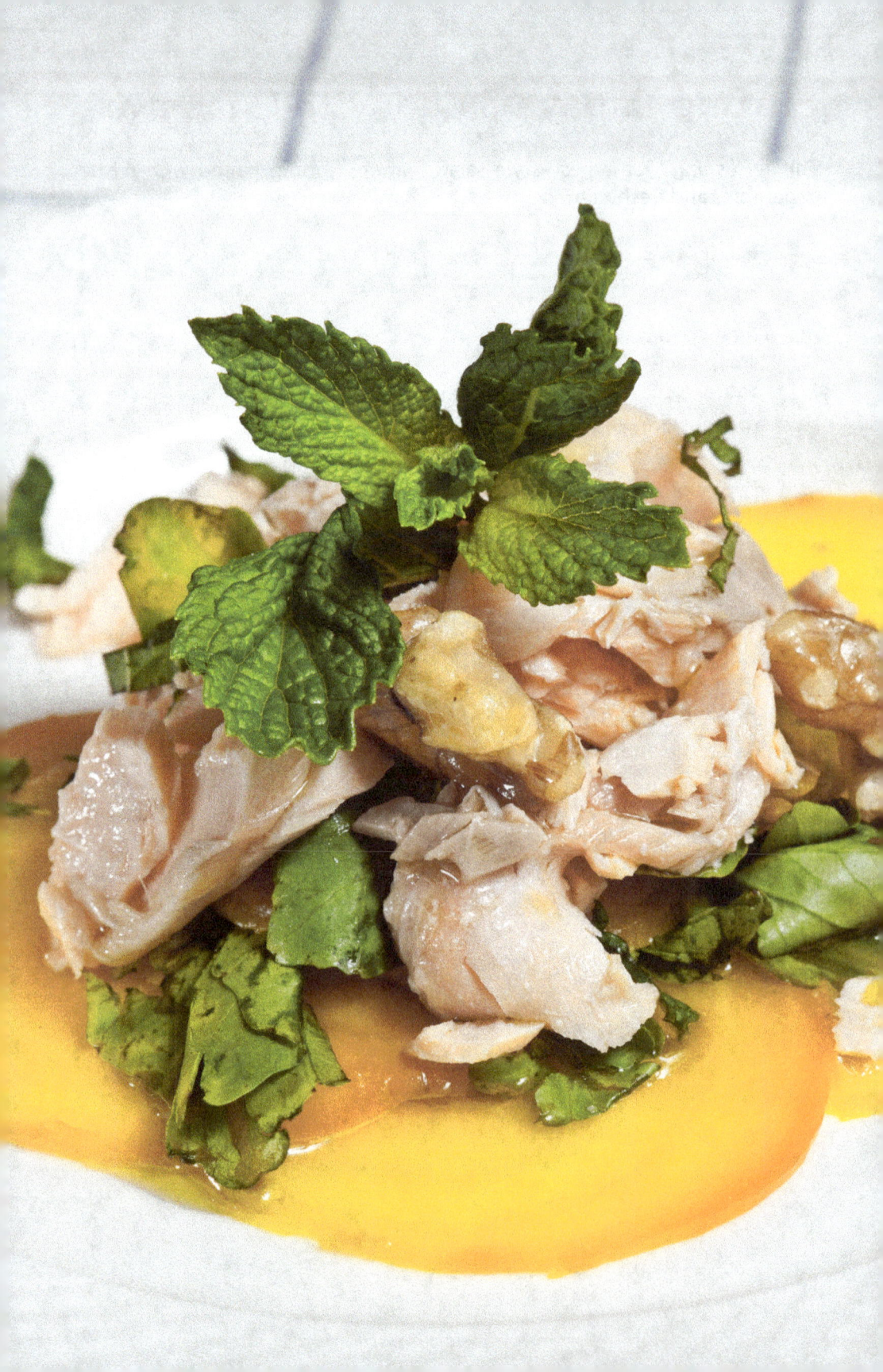

Roasted Beet with Salmon, Walnuts and Mint

Salmon and beets are enlivened with fresh mint. Roast the beet up to one week ahead and peel it just before slicing and serving. The trimmed beet greens are delicious as an addition to soups, or sautéed with garlic and olive oil as a side vegetable.

SERVES 1

- 1 large roasted beet, peeled and thinly sliced
- 1 tbsp. extra virgin olive oil
- 1 tsp. finely chopped shallot
- Pinch dried mustard
- 2 tsps. chopped mint
- 1 tsp. lemon juice
- ½ tsp. grated lemon zest
- 1 large bunch watercress (about ¼ lb.)
- 3–4 oz. cooked salmon filet, crumbled
- 1 tsp. chopped walnuts

Layer the beet slices in an overlapping circle on a plate.

Combine the olive oil, shallot, mustard, mint, lemon juice and lemon zest in a large bowl. Add the watercress and toss to combine. Spoon the watercress into the center of the beets. Sprinkle on the salmon and walnuts and season with freshly ground black pepper to serve.

Chef's Tip: To roast a beet, preheat the oven to 400 degrees F. Trim off the greens and reserve for another use. Wash the beet thoroughly and wrap it (skin on) in foil. Place the beet on a rimmed baking sheet and bake for 1 hour. Allow the beet to cool. Remove the foil and rub the skin off with paper towels. Store in the refrigerator for up to one week.

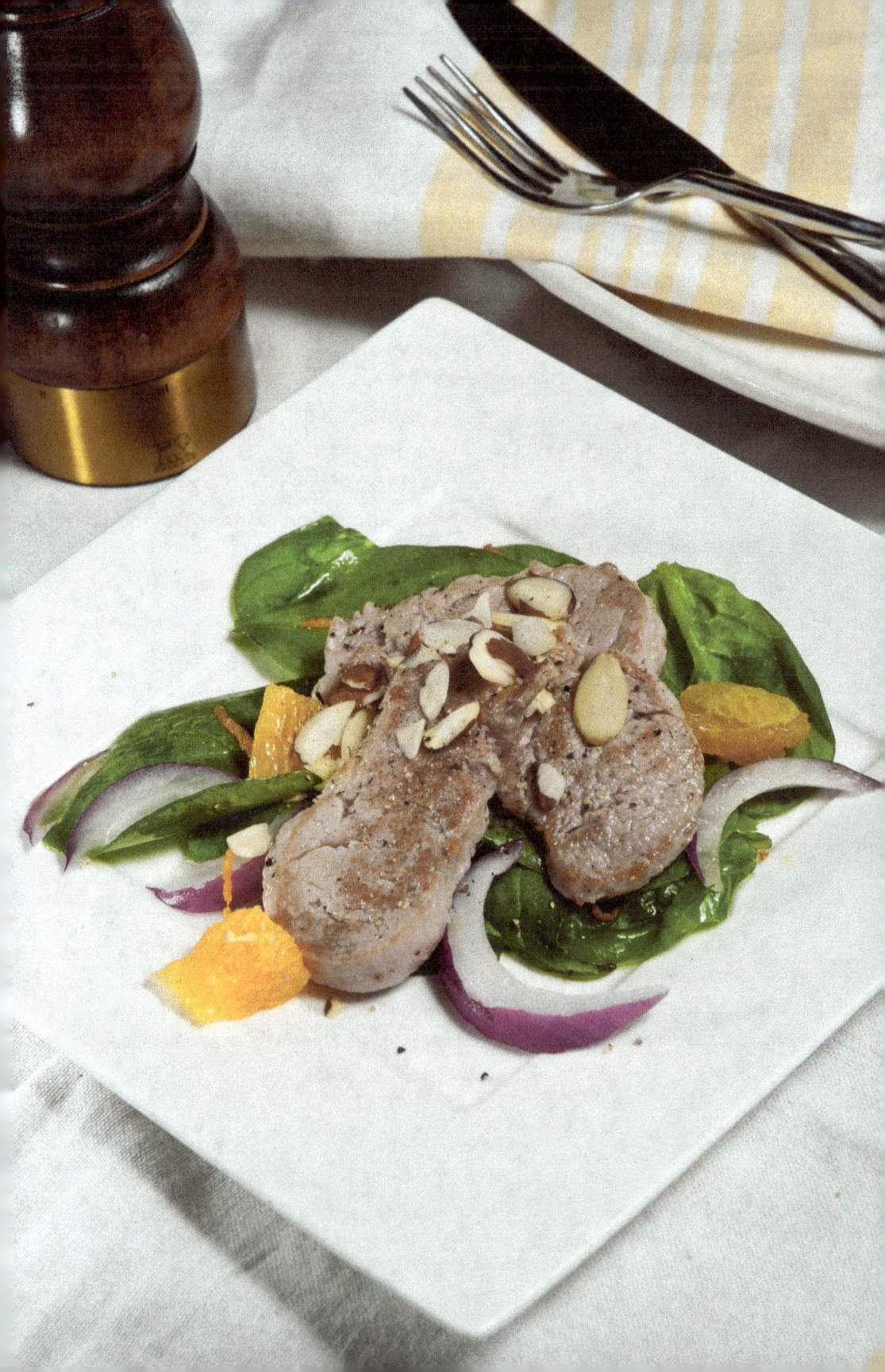

Pork Tenderloin with Spinach, Orange and Onions

Pork tenderloin medallions take minutes to prepare and are a tasty addition to salads. Fresh spinach tossed with orange vinaigrette pairs perfectly with the mustard-seasoned pork.

SERVES 1

- ¼ tsp. dry mustard
- 4 oz. pork tenderloin, thinly sliced into medallions
- 3 tsps. extra virgin olive oil
- 1 tbsp. orange juice
- 1 tsp. orange zest
- 1 ½ cups baby spinach
- ⅛ red onion, thinly sliced
- 3 orange segments, membranes and seeds removed
- 1 tsp. sliced almonds

Sprinkle the mustard evenly onto the pork medallions and season with freshly ground black pepper. Heat 1 tsp. olive oil in a small skillet over medium-high heat. Add the pork in a single layer and cook until lightly browned on the bottom, about 2–3 minutes. Turn the pork and sear until just cooked through, about 1–2 minutes longer. Remove the pork from the skillet and allow to cool.

Whisk together the remaining 2 tsps. oil with the orange juice and zest in a medium bowl. Add the spinach, onion and orange segments and toss to coat. Place the mixture onto a plate and layer on the pork. Sprinkle with the almonds to serve.

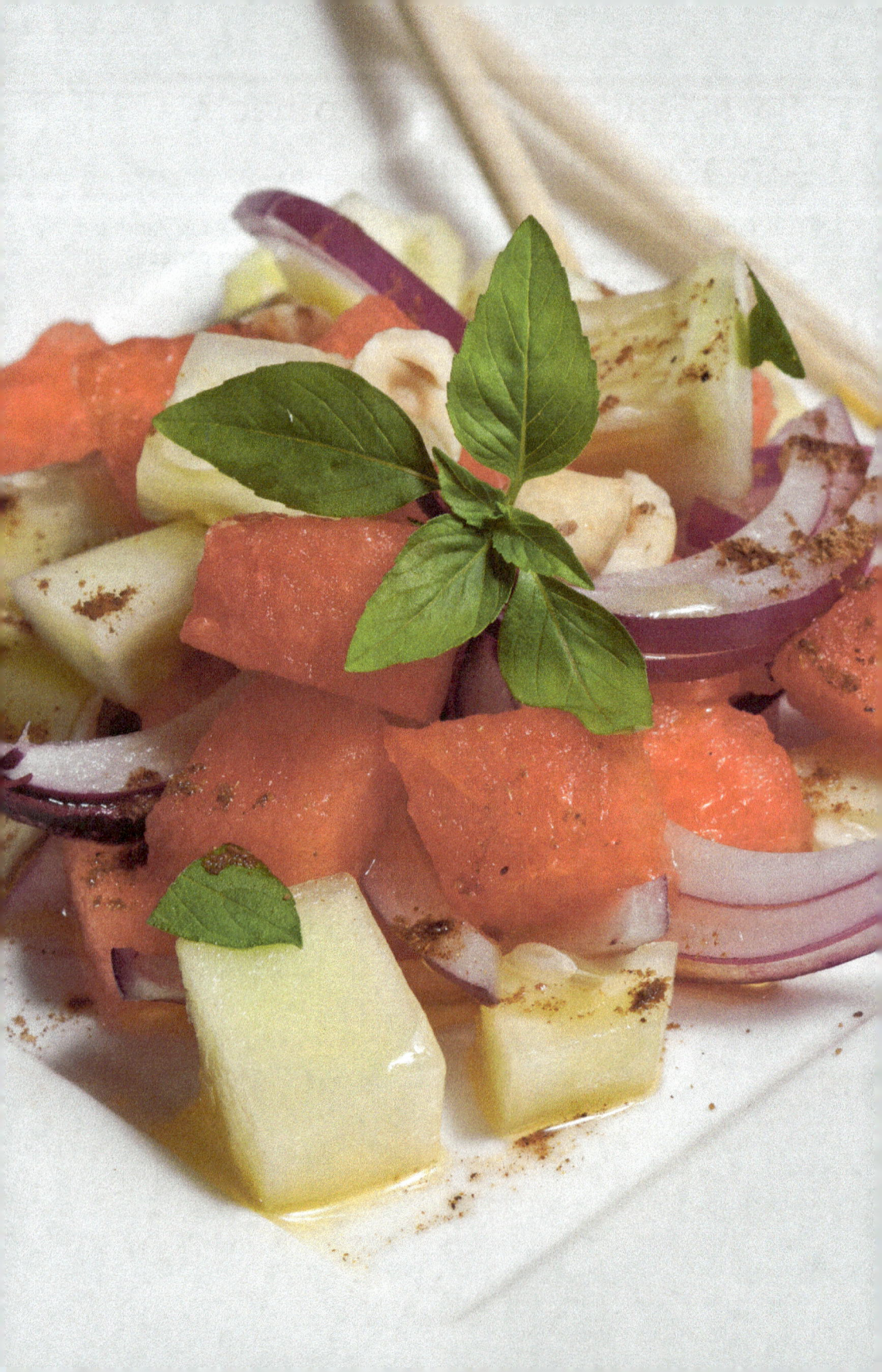

Watermelon, Cucumber and Red Onion with Pork

Thai basil adds a unique licorice accent to this refreshing combination of sweet and savory. If you don't have access to Thai basil, feel free to substitute fresh sweet basil or mint. Cook an extra piece of pork tenderloin when making the dinner on p. 145 to simplify the preparation.

SERVES 1

- 1 tbsp. extra virgin olive oil
- ½ tsp. crushed red pepper
- ¼ tsp. five spice powder
- 1 tsp. lime juice
- 1 tsp. chopped Thai basil
- ½ cup watermelon cubes, diced
- 1 small cucumber, peeled and diced
- ⅛ red onion, thinly sliced (about 2–3 tbsps.)
- 4 oz. cooked pork tenderloin, diced
- 4 toasted hazelnuts, skins removed and coarsely chopped (see Chef's Tip)

Combine the olive oil, red pepper, five spice powder, lime juice and basil in a medium bowl. Add the watermelon, cucumber, red onion and pork and toss to combine. Sprinkle on the hazelnuts to serve.

Chef's Tip: To toast and peel hazelnuts, preheat the oven to 350 degrees F. Spread the hazelnuts in a single layer on a baking sheet and toast them in the oven for about 10–12 minutes, until they've browned a little and the skins are starting to loosen. Carefully wrap the nuts in a kitchen towel and rub vigorously to remove as much loose skin as possible. Let cool completely.

Celery Root, Leek and Pork Belly Soup

Celery root simmered with apple adds rich flavor to this creamy soup. Raw celery root, shaved thin or cut into julienne, also makes a tasty addition to salads.

SERVES 1

- 1 tbsp. extra virgin olive oil
- 1 small leek, trimmed and thinly sliced (about ½ cup)
- 1 medium celery root, peeled and cut into 1" chunks (about 2 cups)
- ½ medium tart apple, peeled, cored and sliced
- ½ tsp. minced garlic
- ¼ tsp. ground coriander
- ¼ tsp. ground cumin
- ¼ tsp. ground turmeric
- ½ tsp. freshly ground pepper
- 1 ½ cups chicken or vegetable stock
- 2 oz. chopped pork belly (see recipe p. 177)

Heat the oil in a medium saucepan or cast-iron Dutch oven over medium heat. Add the leek and sauté until slightly softened, about 4–5 minutes. Add the celery root, apple and garlic and stir to coat. Add the coriander, cumin, turmeric and black pepper. Add the chicken stock and ½ cup water and bring to a boil. Lower the heat to a simmer and cook until the celery root is tender, about 25–30 minutes.

Puree the soup with a blender (or use an immersion blender) until smooth. Sprinkle on the pork belly (if using) and season with freshly ground pepper to serve.

Spicy Chicken Salad with Mustard Greens

This slightly spicy dish is inspired by traditional Thai beef salad, but with the added crunch of peppery mustard greens. Substitute kale or other nutritious greens according to taste and availability. If you haven't prepared the chicken ahead of time while making another meal, see the Chef's Tip on p. 63 for how to poach a chicken breast.

SERVES 1

- 1 tsp. sesame oil
- 2 tsps. coconut oil
- 2 tbsps. chopped red onion
- ½ tsp. crushed red pepper
- 1 tsp. lime juice
- 4 oz. cooked chicken breast, thinly sliced
- 1 scallion, trimmed and thinly sliced lengthwise
- ½ medium cucumber, julienned
- 1 cup mustard greens, ribs removed and cut into ½" strips
- 1 tsp. chopped almonds
- 3 Thai basil leaves, cut into chiffonade (or substitute 2 sweet basil leaves)

Combine the sesame oil, coconut oil, onion, red pepper and lime juice in a medium bowl. Add the chicken, scallion, cucumber and mustard greens and toss to combine. Sprinkle on the almonds and basil to serve.

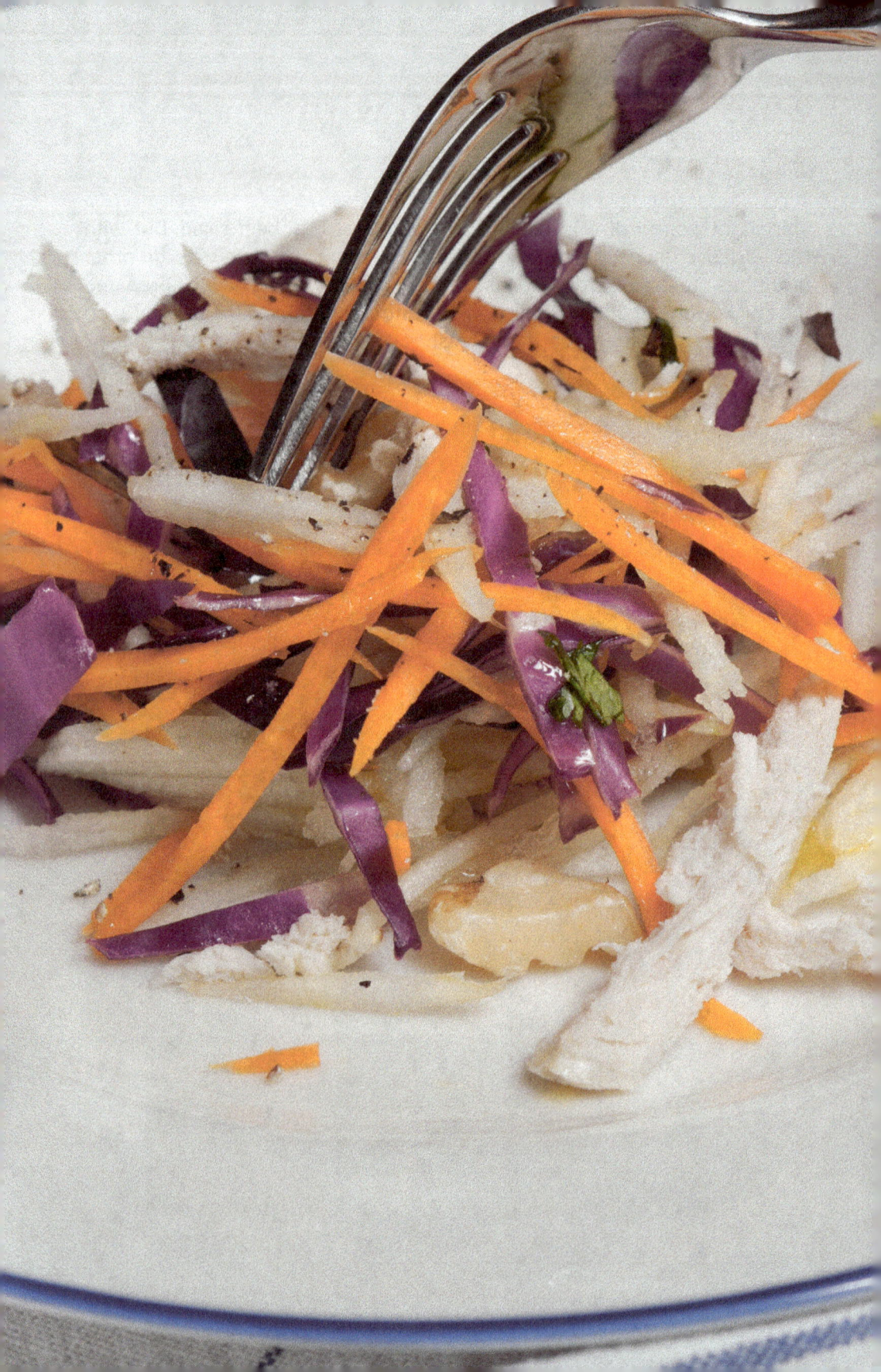

Cabbage, Carrot and Apple Slaw with Chicken

A mixture of textures and flavors come together in this easy-to-prepare dish. If you haven't prepared chicken breast ahead of time as part of another dish, see the Chef's Tip on p. 63 on how to poach a chicken breast.

SERVES 1

- 1 tbsp. avocado oil
- 1 tsp. lime juice
- 1 tsp. chopped fresh thyme
- ½ medium carrot, julienned
- ¼ cup shredded red cabbage
- ½ apple, peeled, seeded and julienned
- 4 oz. cooked chicken breast, shredded
- 1 tbsp. chopped walnuts

Combine the oil, lime juice and thyme in a small bowl. Add the carrot, cabbage, apple and chicken and toss to combine. Season with freshly ground pepper and sprinkle on the walnuts to serve.

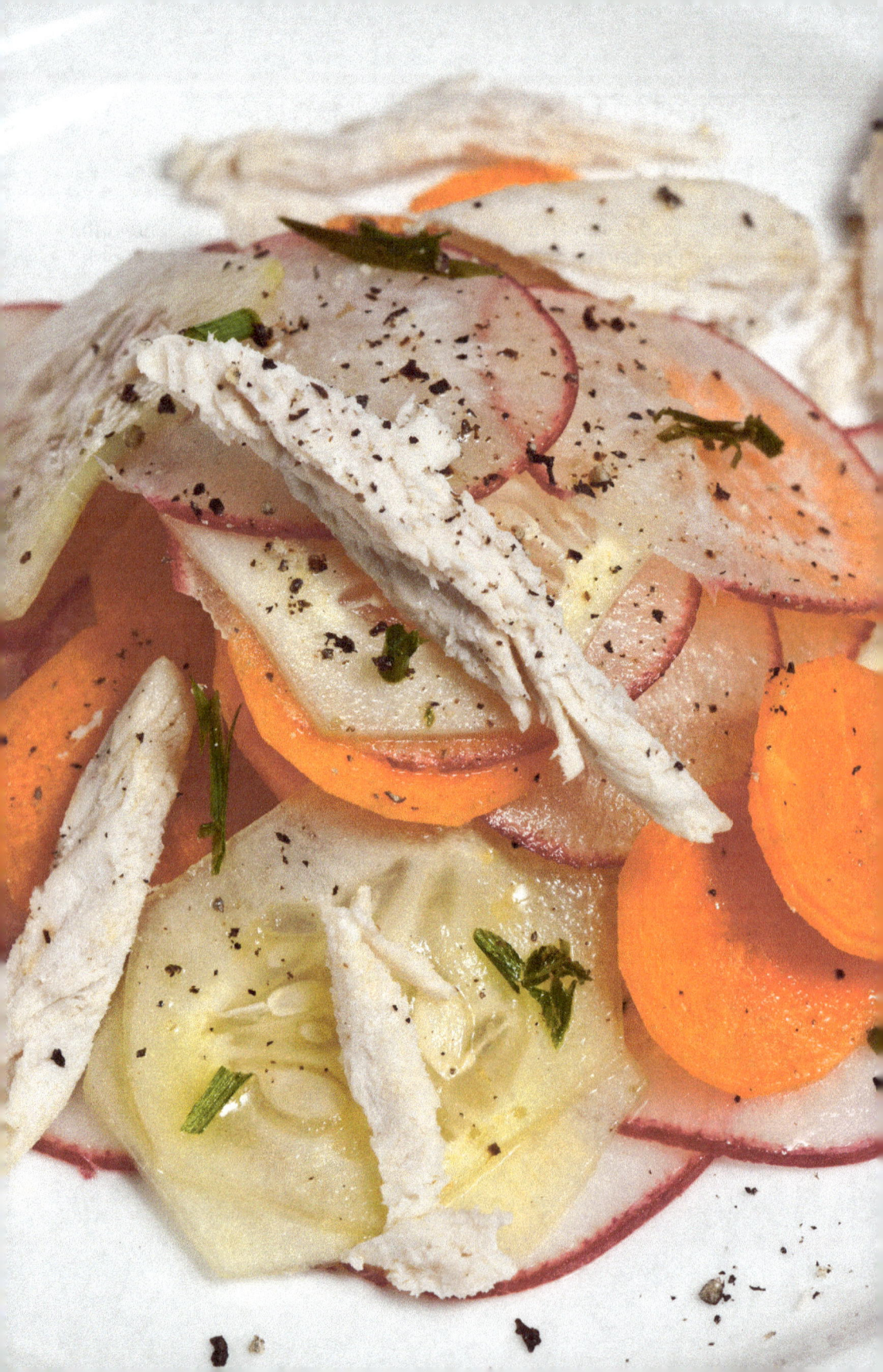

Chicken Salad with Carrot, Radish and Cucumber

Thinly sliced vegetables are the basis for this flavorful chicken salad that tastes as good as it looks. Using a vegetable slicer like a Benriner mandoline makes the preparation quick and easy.

SERVES 1

- 1 tbsp. extra virgin olive oil
- 1 tsp. lemon juice
- 1 tsp. mayonnaise (see recipe p. 163)
- ½ tsp. chopped fresh dill
- ½ medium carrot, trimmed, peeled and sliced paper thin
- 1 medium radish, trimmed and sliced paper thin
- ½ medium cucumber, trimmed and sliced paper thin
- 4 oz. cooked chicken breast, shredded (see Chef's Tip p. 63)
- 1 tsp. chopped chives

Whisk together the olive oil, lemon juice and mayonnaise in a medium bowl until smooth and combined. Stir in the dill. Add the carrot, radish, cucumber and chicken and toss to coat. Sprinkle on the chives and season with pepper to serve.

Spaghetti Squash Primavera with Chicken

Spaghetti squash is often used as a pasta substitute, but its unique texture adds variety to this fresh summery salad. Roast half or all of the spaghetti squash (see Chef's Tip) and reserve the rest for future use, like the lobster dinner on p. 129.

SERVES 1

- 1 tbsp. extra virgin olive oil
- ¼ roasted red pepper, seeded and coarsely chopped
- ½ tsp. dried oregano
- ½ tsp. crushed red pepper
- 1 tsp. lemon juice
- 1 cup cooked spaghetti squash (see Chef's Tip)
- 1 plum tomato, peeled, seeded and coarsely chopped
- ½ medium carrot, peeled and grated
- ¼ cup sliced mushrooms
- ½ cup small broccoli florets, blanched
- 4 oz. cooked shredded chicken breast
- 1 tbsp. chopped flat-leaf parsley
- 1 tsp. toasted pine nuts

Combine the olive oil, roasted pepper, oregano and crushed red pepper in a medium bowl. Stir in the lemon juice. Add the spaghetti squash and toss to combine.

Add the tomato, carrot, mushrooms, broccoli and chicken and toss to coat. Season with freshly ground pepper. Sprinkle on the parsley and pine nuts to serve.

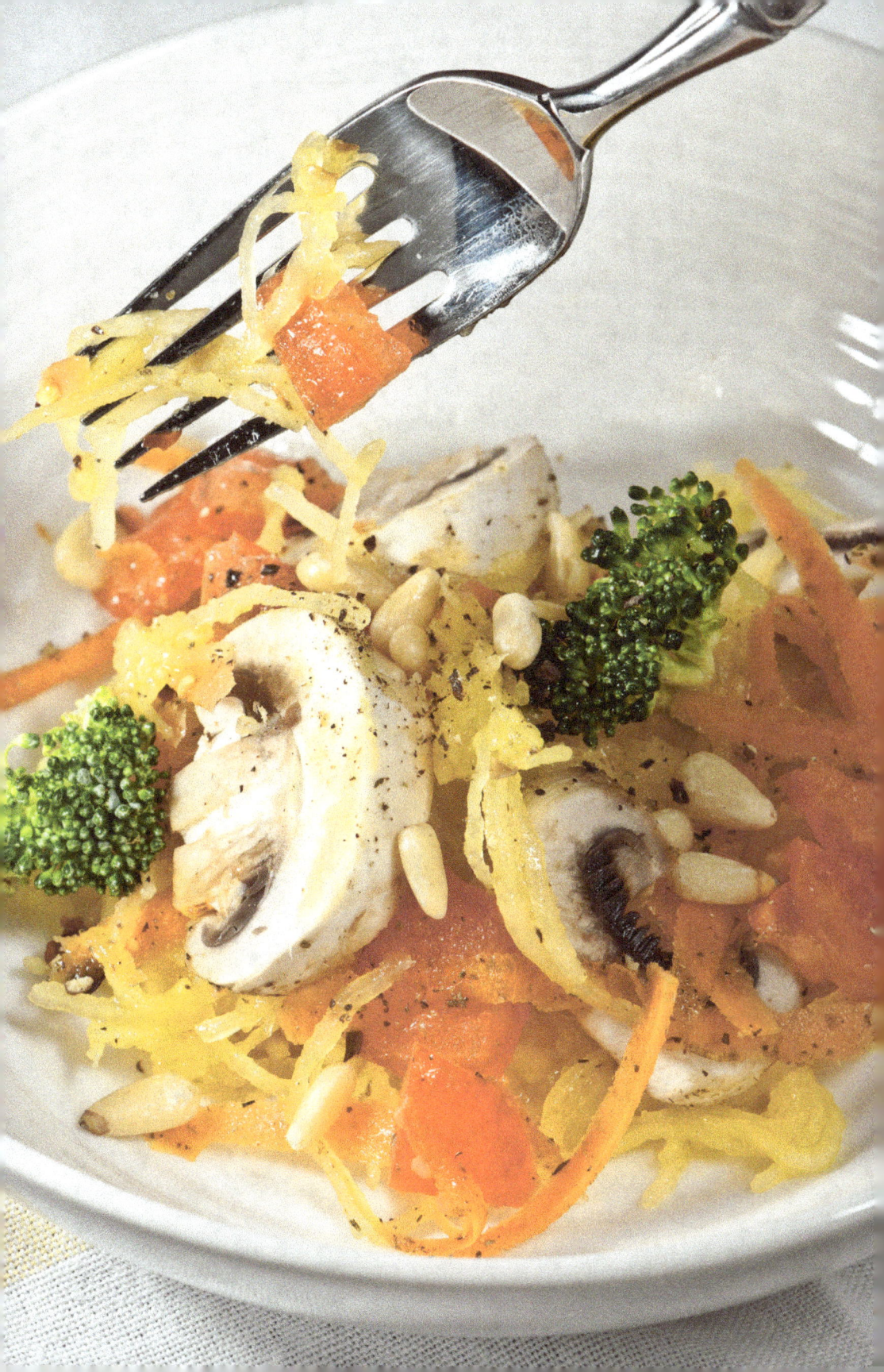

Chef's Tip: To roast the spaghetti squash, preheat the oven to 400 degrees F. Line a baking dish with foil. Cut the squash in half and remove and discard the seeds. Place the squash cut side down on the baking sheet and add about 1" water to the pan. Prick the skin of the squash with a fork. Cover with foil and bake for 30–35 minutes until just tender. Remove from the oven and let rest until cool enough to handle. Scrape the strands of squash from inside of the skin with a fork and discard the skin. If using for a salad, refrigerate covered until completely chilled through. A small (4–5 lb.) squash yields about 2 ½ cups.

Chicken and Coconut Soup with Cauliflower

The addition of cauliflower to this traditional Thai-style soup adds texture and fiber for a filling dish. Fresh and frozen kaffir lime leaves are available at Asian groceries. If unavailable, substitute the dried leaves available in the spice section of many conventional markets.

SERVES 1

- ½ cup coconut milk (about ⅓ can)
- ½ cup chicken stock
- 1 lemon grass stalk, trimmed and coarsely chopped
- 1 kaffir lime leaf, thinly sliced
- 1 Thai chili pepper, seeded and sliced in half
- 1 thin slice ginger
- 2 black peppercorns
- 4 oz. boneless, skinless chicken breast, cut into thin strips
- 8 white mushrooms, cut in half
- ½ cup cauliflower florets
- 1 tbsp. lime juice
- 1 scallion, trimmed and coarsely chopped
- 1 tsp. chopped fresh cilantro

Combine the coconut milk and chicken stock in a medium saucepan and bring to a boil. Add the lemon grass, kaffir lime leaf, chili pepper, ginger and peppercorns. Lower the heat and simmer for 10 minutes, to infuse the flavors into the soup base. Strain the liquid into a clean medium saucepan and discard the seasonings.

Bring the soup to a simmer over low and add the chicken and mushrooms. Cook for 3 minutes. Add the cauliflower and cook for 3-4 minutes longer, until the chicken is cooked through and the cauliflower is just tender. Remove from the heat and stir in the lime juice, scallion and cilantro to serve.

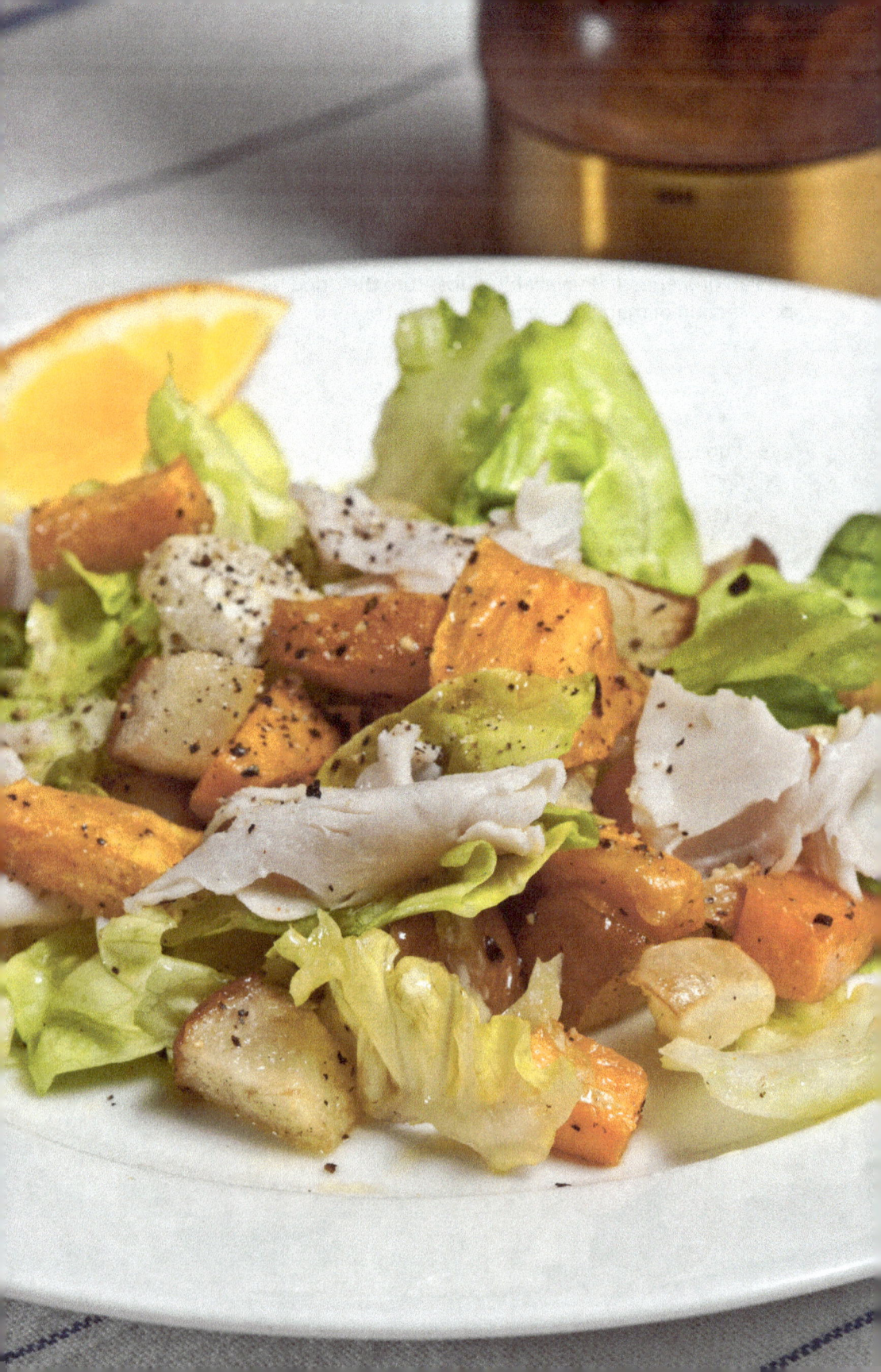

Turkey with Roasted Sweet Potato, Turnip and Pear

Roast the vegetables and fruit ahead of time while roasting other items to reduce the preparation time for this tasty salad. The easy-to-make Moroccan seasoning adds exotic flavor.

SERVES 1

- ¼ sweet potato, cut into ¾" cubes
- ½ medium turnip, trimmed and cut into ¾" cubes
- ½ medium pear, seeded, trimmed and cut into ¾" cubes
- 1 ½ tbsps. extra virgin olive oil
- ½ tsp. dried thyme
- 1 tsp. Moroccan Spice Blend (see recipe p. 161)
- 1 tbsp. orange juice
- ½ tsp. finely grated orange zest
- 1 cup spring mix or other tender lettuce
- 4 oz. cooked turkey breast or cutlet, thinly sliced

Preheat the oven to 450 degrees F. Lightly grease a baking sheet.

Combine the sweet potato, turnip and pear in a medium bowl. Toss the mixture with ½ tbsp. olive oil and sprinkle on the thyme and Moroccan spice. Place the mixture in a single layer on the baking sheet. Roast until tender and lightly browned, about 20–25 minutes. Allow the vegetables to cool completely.

Combine the remaining 1 tbsp. olive oil with the orange juice and zest in a medium bowl. Add the roasted vegetables and pear, and toss to coat. Add the lettuce and turkey breast and toss to combine. Season with freshly ground black pepper to serve.

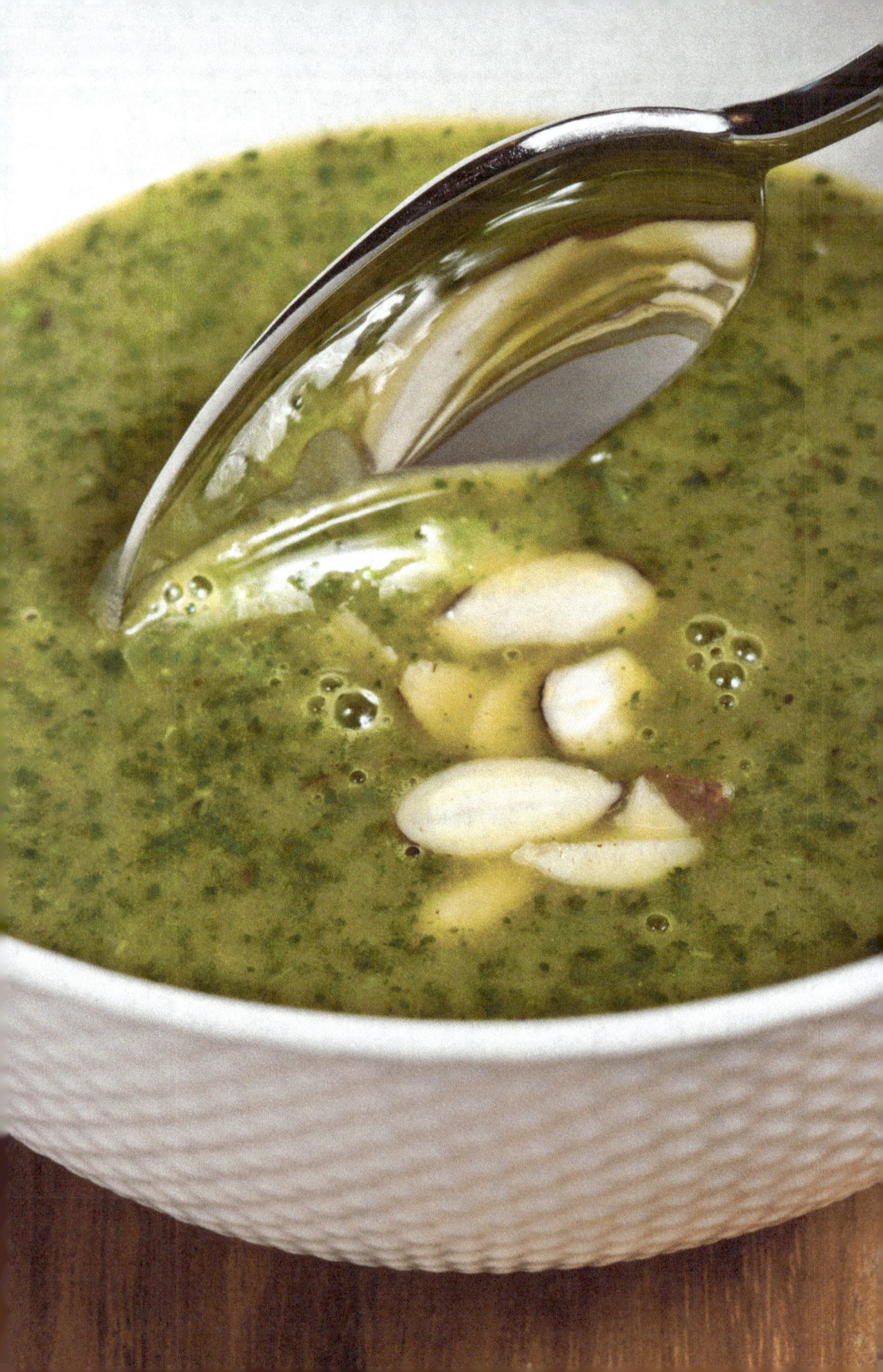

Watercress and Sweet Potato Soup

Watercress adds a rich, peppery flavor to this delicious soup. Remove and discard the large stems from the watercress, but cook and puree the smaller ones along with the leaves. Add shredded chicken or pork for a more substantial dish.

SERVES 1

- 1 tbsp. extra virgin olive oil
- 2 tbsps. chopped onion
- ¼ tsp. minced garlic
- ½ medium sweet potato, peeled and diced
- 2 cups vegetable or chicken stock
- ½ tsp. crushed red pepper
- ½ tsp. five spice powder
- 1 large bunch watercress (about ¼ lb.)
- 1 tsp. lime juice
- 1 tsp. sliced almonds

Heat the olive oil in a medium saucepan or cast-iron Dutch oven. Add the onion and cook until softened, about 4–5 minutes. Add the garlic and cook for 30 seconds. Add the sweet potato, 1 ½ cups stock and 1 cup water. Bring to a boil and lower the heat to a simmer. Stir in the red pepper and five spice powder. Simmer until the sweet potato is very soft, about 20–25 minutes.

Add the watercress and cook for 5 minutes longer. Remove from the heat and stir in the remaining ½ cup stock.

Puree the mixture with a blender (or use an immersion blender) until smooth. Reheat the soup and season with freshly ground pepper to taste. Stir in the lime juice and sprinkle on the almonds to serve.

Curried Zucchini Spinach Soup

This soup is delicious served warm or chilled. Add crabmeat or cooked shrimp for a more substantial meal.

SERVES 1

- 2 tsps. extra virgin olive oil
- 3 tbsps. chopped onion
- ¼ tsp. minced garlic
- ¼ tsp. ground cumin
- ¼ tsp. ground coriander
- ¼ tsp. chili powder
- Pinch ground cloves
- 2 cups chicken or vegetable stock
- 1 medium zucchini, trimmed and coarsely chopped (about 1 ½–2 cups)
- 1 cup baby spinach
- 1 tsp. lemon juice
- Freshly ground pepper
- 3 cherry tomatoes, coarsely chopped
- 1 scallion, trimmed and coarsely chopped

Set a large bowl in an ice bath.

Heat the oil in a medium saucepan or Dutch oven over medium heat. Add the chopped onion and sauté until softened, about 4–5 minutes. Add the garlic and sauté for 30 seconds more. Stir in the cumin, coriander, chili powder and cloves. Add the stock and bring to a boil. Add the zucchini and cook until tender, about 4–5 minutes. Add the spinach and parsley and stir for 30 seconds, until spinach is just wilted. Immediately remove from the heat and pour the mixture into the chilled bowl. Stir the mixture to cool it quickly. Stir in the lemon juice.

Puree the mixture in a blender (or use an immersion blender) until smooth. Strain the mixture through a fine sieve and season with pepper. If serving chilled, refrigerate for at least 2 hours. If serving warm, heat the mixture in a medium saucepan over medium until heated through. Garnish with the tomatoes and scallion to serve.

Wild Mushroom Soup

Dried porcini mushrooms add a rich, woodsy flavor to this elegant soup. The soup has a meaty texture, but becomes a more substantial meal with the addition of shredded pork or short-ribs.

SERVES 1

- 1–2 dried porcini mushrooms (or substitute other dried wild mushrooms, about ⅛ oz.)
- 1 tbsp. extra virgin olive oil
- 2 tbsps. chopped onion
- 1 leek, white part only, trimmed, cleaned and finely chopped
- ½ tsp. minced garlic
- ½ celery stalk, trimmed and finely chopped
- 1 ½ cups sliced fresh wild mushrooms like chanterelles (or substitute shitakes)
- 2 cups chicken stock or vegetable stock
- 1 bay leaf
- 1 thyme sprig
- 1 tsp. chopped flat-leaf parsley

Place the dried porcini in a bowl or measuring cup and cover with ½ cup boiling water. Allow the mushrooms to soak for 30 minutes. Line a strainer with cheesecloth and set it over a bowl. Drain the porcinis through the strainer. Squeeze the mushrooms over the strainer to extract as much flavorful liquid as possible. Coarsely chop the mushrooms and rinse them several times to remove any sand.

Heat the olive oil over medium heat in a medium saucepan or cast-iron Dutch oven. Add the onion and leek. Cook until softened, about 4–5 minutes. Add the garlic and celery and cook for 30 seconds. Add the fresh and reconstituted mushrooms and cook until softened, about 4–5 minutes.

Add the reserved mushroom water, stock, bay leaf and thyme sprig and bring to a boil over medium-high heat. Reduce the heat, cover and simmer for 45 minutes. Remove and discard the bay leaf and thyme. Allow to cool slightly.

Puree the soup with a blender (or use an immersion blender) until smooth. Return to the pot and add freshly ground pepper to taste. Sprinkle on the parsley to serve.

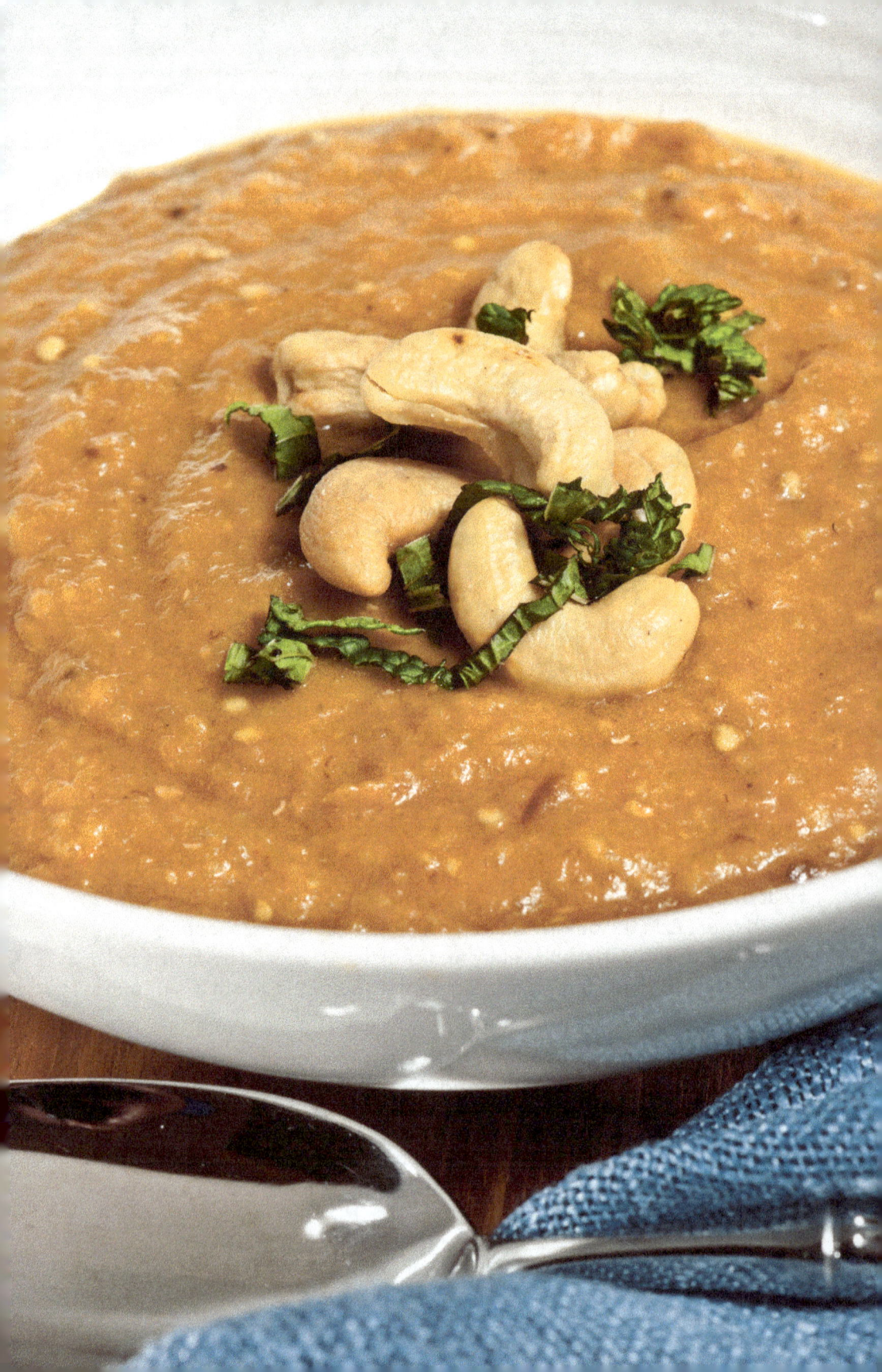

Roasted Eggplant and Tomato Soup

Roasting the vegetables adds rich flavor to this savory soup. Add shredded chicken or pork for a more substantial dish.

SERVES 1

- ¼ large eggplant, peeled and cut into ½" cubes
- ¼ medium onion, thinly sliced
- 1 tbsp. extra virgin olive oil
- ½ tsp. thyme leaves
- 1 medium slicing tomato, cored and cut into quarters
- 1 ½ cups chicken or vegetable stock
- ½ tsp. smoked paprika
- ¼ tsp. ground cumin
- ¼ tsp. ground coriander
- 1 tsp. lime juice
- 1 tsp. chopped flat-leaf parsley
- 4-6 cashews

Preheat the oven to 400 degrees F. Line a rimmed baking sheet with foil.

Place the eggplant and onion in a medium bowl. Drizzle on ½ tbsp. olive oil and thyme and toss to coat. Spread the eggplant mixture in a single layer on the baking sheet. Drizzle the remaining ½ tbsp. olive oil onto the tomato quarters and place them onto the baking sheet. Roast for 20–25 minutes, until the vegetables are tender and lightly browned and softened. Remove and discard the skin and seeds from the tomato.

Place the vegetables in a medium saucepan or a cast-iron Dutch oven and add the stock, smoked paprika, cumin and coriander. Bring to a boil over medium-high heat. Lower to a simmer and cook until vegetables are very tender, about 10–12 minutes.

Puree the mixture in a blender (or use an immersion blender) until smooth. Strain the soup through a fine mesh sieve if a smoother texture is desired. Stir in the lime juice and season with freshly ground pepper. Sprinkle on the parsley and cashews to serve.

Spicy Sweet Potato and Parsnip Soup

This hearty blend of vegetables is seasoned with Middle Eastern spices and pureed into a creamy soup. Add cooked ground pork or turkey for a more substantial meal.

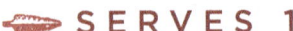 **SERVES 1**

- 1 tbsp. extra virgin olive oil
- 1 ½ tsps. Moroccan Spice Blend (see recipe p. 161)
- ½ crushed red pepper
- 3 tbsps. chopped onion
- ¼ butternut squash, peeled and cut into cubes (about 1 cup cubes)
- 1 medium parsnip, trimmed, peeled and cut into 1" dice
- ½ medium sweet potato, peeled and cut into 1" cubes
- 1 cup chicken stock
- ½ medium apple, peeled, seeded and diced
- 1 tsp. lime juice
- 1 tsp. chopped flat-leaf parsley
- 1 tsp. toasted pumpkin seeds

Heat the olive oil in a medium saucepan or cast-iron Dutch oven over medium heat. Add the spice blend and sauté for 30 seconds. Add the red pepper, onion, squash, parsnip and sweet potato and sauté for 1 minute. Stir in the chicken stock and ½ cup water and bring to a boil. Lower to a simmer and cook until the vegetables are tender, about 20–25 minutes.

Add the apple and remove from the heat. Allow the mixture to cool slightly and puree with an immersion blender (or use a blender) until smooth. Stir in the lime juice and garnish with the chopped parsley and pumpkin seeds to serve.

CHAPTER THREE
25 Dinners

- Spicy Lamb Burger with Orange Herb Slaw
- Lamb Tagine with Star Anise
- Meatloaf with Roasted Red Pepper and Cauliflower
- Filet Mignon with Celery Root and Mushrooms
- Veal Chop with Broccoli Rabe
- Chili and Mint Fish Cake with Broccoli Puree
- Sesame Shrimp with Orange and Almonds
- Lobster with Arugula and Spaghetti Squash
- Sea Scallops with Cherry Tomatoes, Avocado and Macadamias
- Pan-Seared Tuna with Caramelized Onions and Mango Salsa
- Moroccan Fish Stew
- Mediterranean Halibut in Parchment
- Trout with Carrot and Walnuts
- Salmon with Red Cabbage, Brussels Sprouts and Hazelnuts
- Pan-Roasted Mussels with Onions and Basil
- Red Snapper with Leeks and Saffron
- Pork Ribs with Jicama Slaw
- Pork Loin Chop with Peaches, Squash and Pecans
- Pork Tenderloin with Cherries and Kale
- Five Spice Chicken with Tangerine and Fennel

- Chicken with Pesto and Cauliflower Puree
- Zucchini-Stuffed Game Hen with Turnip and Mushrooms
- Beet and Parsnip Chips with Shredded Chicken
- Green Coconut Curry with Chicken and Cabbage
- Turkey, Zucchini and Butternut Squash Strata

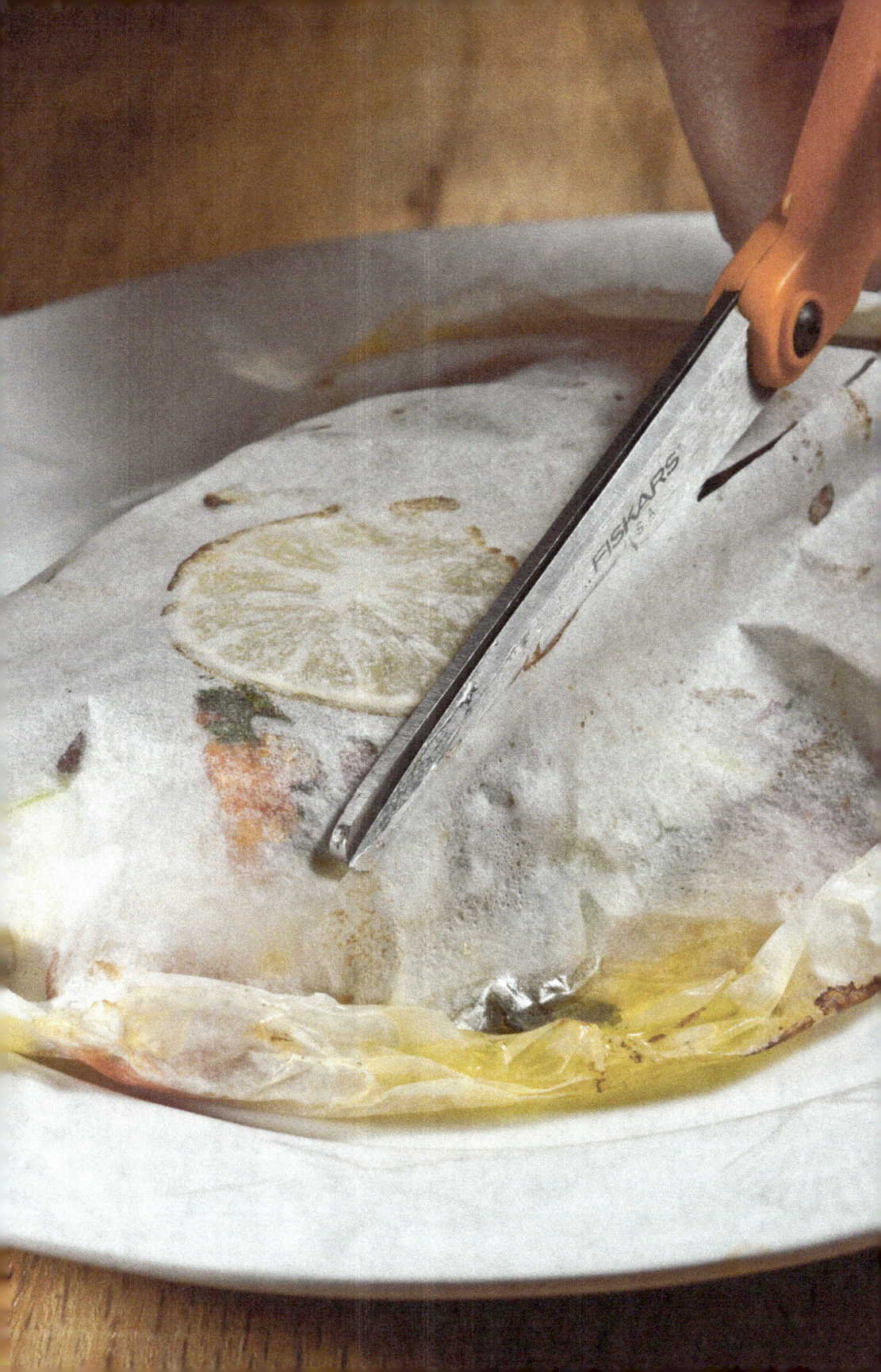

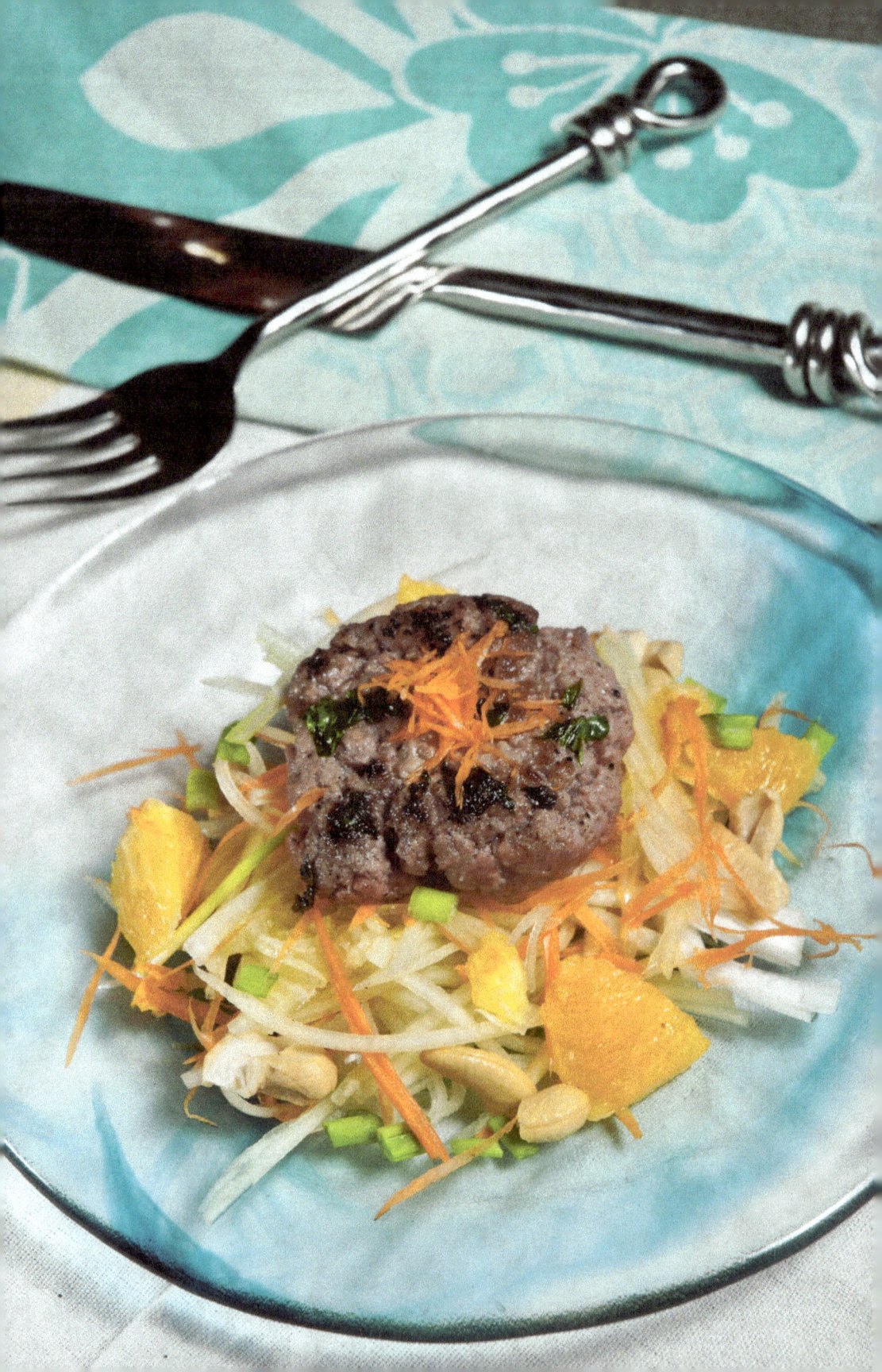

Spicy Lamb Burger with Orange Herb Slaw

This seasoned lamb burger is also delicious with the added flavor of the grill.

SERVES 1

- 1 tbsp. extra virgin olive oil
- 1 tsp. orange juice
- 1 tsp. orange zest
- ½ tsp. chopped basil
- ½ tsp. chopped flat-leaf parsley
- 4 orange segments, peeled, seeded and chopped
- 1 scallion, trimmed and thinly sliced lengthwise
- ½ carrot, peeled and julienned
- ½ cucumber, peeled, seeded and julienned
- 1 tsp. minced garlic
- ½ tsp. crushed red pepper
- ½ tsp. chili powder
- 1 tsp. chopped fresh mint
- 1 tbsp. chopped red onion
- ½ tsp. lime juice
- 4 oz. ground lamb
- 4 large cashews, coarsely chopped

Whisk together the olive oil and orange juice in a medium bowl. Add the orange zest, basil, parsley and orange segments and stir to combine. Add the scallion, carrot and cucumber and toss to coat. Cover and refrigerate for 20 minutes.

In the meantime, preheat the broiler and set the rack 3-4 inches from the heat.

Combine the garlic, pepper, chili powder, mint, onion and lime juice in a small bowl. Add the lamb and mix thoroughly. Form the lamb into a patty about ½" thick. Place the patty on a broiler pan and broil for 2 minutes. Turn the burger and broil for 2-3 minutes longer for medium-rare (or according to desired degree of doneness). Season the slaw with freshly ground pepper and serve with the lamb burger.

Lamb Tagine with Star Anise

A tagine is a traditional North African dish similar to a stew in that it cooks in a single pot (which is also called a tagine). In this version, lamb is cooked until tender in a lightly seasoned tomato broth flavored with star anise.

SERVES 1

- ¼ tsp. dry mustard
- 1 tsp. Moroccan Spice Blend (see recipe p. 161)
- ¼ tsp. freshly ground black pepper
- 1 (6–8 oz.) lamb shoulder chop or 2 (4 oz.) lamb loin chops
- 1 tbsp. extra virgin olive oil
- 3 tbsps. coarsely chopped onion
- ½ carrot, peeled and coarsely chopped
- ½ celery stalk, coarsely chopped
- 1 tsp. finely minced ginger
- ¼ cup orange juice
- 2 plum tomatoes, seeded and coarsely chopped
- 1 ½ cups chicken or vegetable stock
- 1 star anise
- 1 cup broccoli florets, blanched
- 1 tsp. chopped fresh mint

Combine the mustard, Moroccan spice and pepper in a small bowl. Sprinkle the mixture evenly over the lamb chop.

Heat the oil in a medium saucepan or cast-iron Dutch oven over medium-high heat. Add the lamb chop and cook until lightly browned on both sides, about 3–4 minutes per side. Remove from the pan and set aside. Add the onion, carrot, celery and ginger to the pan and cook until the onion is softened, about 4–5 minutes. Add the orange juice and scrape up any bits off the bottom of the pan. Add the tomatoes, stock, ¼ cup water and star anise and bring to a boil. Lower the heat and add the lamb chop. Simmer for 1 hour, until lamb is tender, adding a little extra stock as necessary.

Remove the chop to a cutting board. Remove and discard the star anise. Cut off all the meat and return it to the sauce.

Stir in the broccoli and cook for 3–4 minutes, until just tender. Remove from the heat and stir in the mint to serve.

Meatloaf with Roasted Red Pepper and Cauliflower

This pistachio-studded meatloaf is served with roasted cauliflower glazed with roasted red pepper. It may also be made with ground bison. Because it makes a single serving, it bakes more quickly than typical recipes. If you increase the serving size (the meatloaf is also delicious cold), increase the cooking time by 10–15 minutes for each additional serving.

SERVES 1

- 2 tsps. extra virgin olive oil
- 1 tbsp. minced onion
- ¼ cup chopped mushrooms
- ¼ tsp. minced garlic
- 1 cup cauliflower florets
- 1 large egg
- 1 tsp. chopped fresh flat-leaf parsley
- ½ tsp. smoked paprika
- 2 oz. ground beef
- 2 oz. ground veal
- 2 oz. ground pork
- 1 tsp. chopped pistachios
- 3 tbsp. coconut milk
- ½ roasted red pepper, seeded and chopped
- ½ tsp. crushed red pepper
- 1 tsp. sesame seeds

Preheat oven to 425 degrees F. Lightly grease a small mini-loaf pan or individual ramekin. Cover a rimmed baking sheet with aluminum foil.

Heat 1 tsp. olive oil in a small skillet over medium heat. Add the onion and mushrooms and cook until just softened, about 3–4 minutes. Stir in the garlic and cook for 30 seconds longer. Allow the mixture to cool.

In the meantime, toss the cauliflower with the remaining 1 tsp. olive oil and season with freshly ground pepper. Spread the cauliflower in a single layer on the baking sheet. Roast until just tender and edges are golden brown, about 18–20 minutes. Set aside.

Whisk the egg in a medium bowl. Divide the whisked egg in half and reserve half for another use. Stir in the onion/mushroom mixture, parsley and smoked paprika. Add the ground beef, veal, pork and pistachios and mix to combine. Press the mixture into the loaf pan and bake for 25–30 minutes, until lightly browned and cooked through (internal temperature should read 160 degrees F).

Combine the coconut milk and roasted pepper with a food processor or blender until smooth. Stir in the crushed red pepper and sesame seeds. Heat the mixture in a small saucepan over medium heat. Add the cauliflower and stir until just heated through.

Spoon the cauliflower mixture onto a plate and place the meatloaf next to it. Season with pepper to serve.

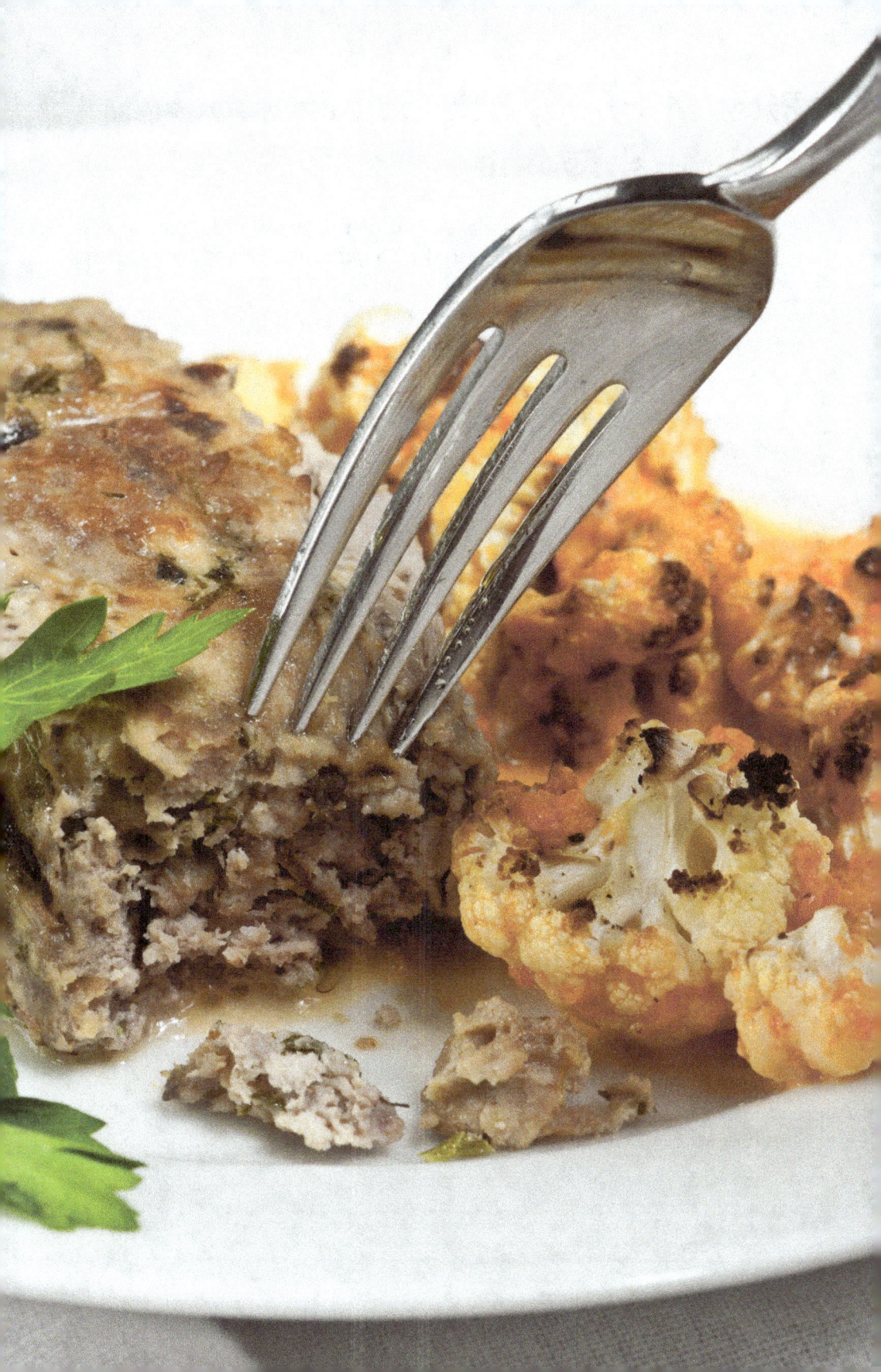

Filet Mignon with Celery Root and Mushrooms

Filet mignon is cut from the smaller end of the beef tenderloin, so it is typically very tender. Here it is roasted with garlic and served over creamy celery root puree with a rich mushroom sauce.

SERVES 1

- 2 tbsps. coconut milk
- 5 tbsps. chicken stock
- ¼ lb. celery root, peeled and coarsely chopped (about ½ cup)
- 1 tsp. coconut oil
- Pinch cayenne pepper
- 1 tsp. chopped flat-leaf parsley
- 4–6 oz. filet mignon
- 1 clove garlic, peeled and thinly sliced
- 1 tbsp. extra virgin olive oil
- 1 tsp. minced shallot
- ¼ cup sliced shitake mushrooms
- ¼ tsp. minced fresh rosemary
- ½ tsp. lemon juice

Combine the coconut milk, 2 tbsps. chicken stock, ½ cup water and celery root in a small saucepan. Bring to a boil over medium-high heat. Lower the heat and simmer until tender, about 20–25 minutes. Pour off and discard all but 1 tbsp. excess liquid. Puree with a blender (or use an immersion blender) until smooth. Add the coconut oil, cayenne pepper and parsley and blend to combine. Set aside and keep warm.

In the meantime, preheat the oven to 400 degrees F. Lightly grease a small baking dish or roasting pan.

Season the filet generously with freshly ground pepper. Using a paring knife, make 5-6 small slits (about ½" deep) around the circumference of the steak and insert a slice of garlic into each slit. Heat ½ tbsp. olive oil in a small skillet (preferably cast-iron) over medium-high heat. Add the filet and brown on all sides, about 3-4 minutes.

Transfer to the baking dish and roast for 6–7 minutes for medium-rare (to an internal temperature of 140–145 degrees F), or until desired degree of doneness. Loosely cover the steak with foil and allow it to rest for 5 minutes.

In the same skillet used for the steak, heat the remaining ½ tbsp. olive oil over medium-high heat. Add the shallot and mushrooms and season with freshly ground pepper. Cook until the mushrooms are softened, about 6–7 minutes. Add the remaining 3 tbsps. stock and rosemary, scraping up any brown bits from the bottom of the pan. Simmer until half the liquid has evaporated, about 3–4 minutes, and remove from the heat. Stir in the lemon juice.

Spoon the celery root puree onto a plate. Set the steak on top and spoon on the mushroom sauce to serve.

Veal Chop with Broccoli Rabe

This Tuscan-inspired veal chop is finished with lemon zest and olive oil and served over a bed of delicious sautéed greens studded with walnuts.

SERVES 1

- 1 ½ tbsps. extra virgin olive oil
- 1 (8–10 oz.) veal rib chop (about ¾" thick)
- ¼ tsp. garlic
- ½ tsp. crushed red pepper
- ½ bunch broccoli rabe (about ¼ lb.), blanched (see Chef's Tip)
- ⅓ cup chicken or vegetable stock
- 1 tsp. chopped walnuts
- 1 tsp. lemon juice
- 1 tbsp. fresh chopped parsley
- ½ tsp. lemon zest

Preheat the oven to 400 degrees F. Lightly grease a small baking dish or roasting pan.

Heat ½ tbsp. olive oil in a medium skillet. Season the veal chop with pepper and add to the pan. Cook, turning once, until golden brown, about 3-4 minutes per side. Remove the chop from the pan to the baking dish and roast for 6-8 minutes for medium-rare (internal temperature of 145 degrees F) or to desired degree of doneness. Remove from the oven and cover loosely with foil to keep warm.

In the meantime, return the skillet to medium heat and add ½ tbsp. olive oil. Add the garlic and red pepper and cook for 30 seconds. Add the broccoli rabe and cook for 30 seconds. Add the chicken stock and bring to a boil. Lower the heat to a simmer. Cover and cook until tender, stirring occasionally, about 5-7 minutes. Stir in the walnuts and keep warm.

Spoon the broccoli rabe onto a plate and top with the veal chop. Drizzle the remaining ½ tbsp. olive oil over the veal chop. Sprinkle the lemon juice, parsley and lemon zest evenly over the veal and broccoli rabe to serve.

Chef's Tip: To blanch the broccoli rabe, first remove and discard the larger stems. Fill a medium bowl about halfway with ice and then fill with water. Fill a medium saucepan with water and bring to a boil over high heat. Add the broccoli rabe and allow the water to return to a boil. Cook for 3 minutes, until bright green and slightly tender. Pour the broccoli rabe into a metal strainer to drain off the water and immediately plunge it into the ice bath. When completely chilled through, drain the broccoli rabe and press with paper towels to remove any excess water.

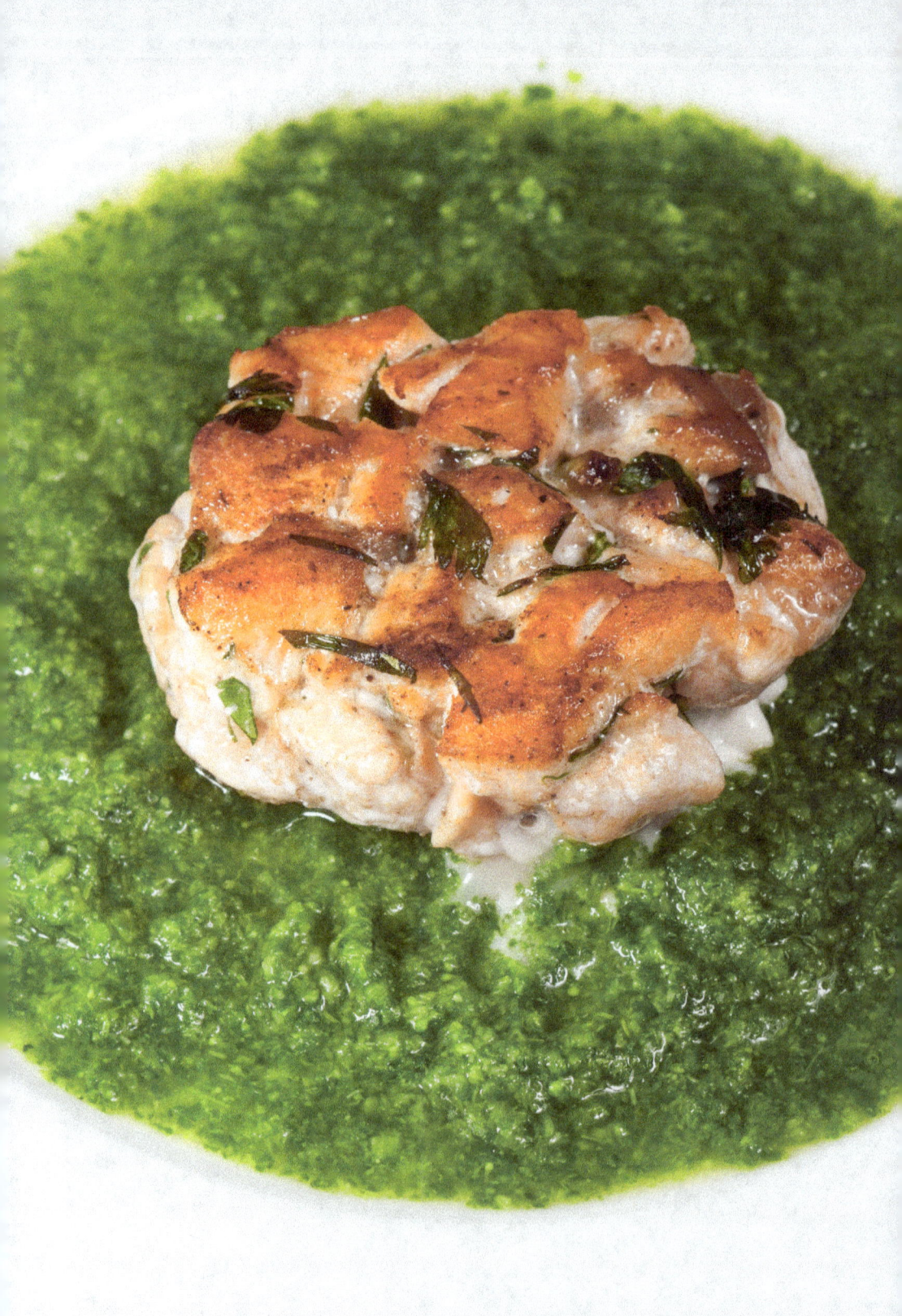

Chili and Mint Fish Cake with Broccoli Puree

This Vietnamese-inspired fish cake is served over a smooth broccoli and spinach puree for a sophisticated dish.

SERVES 1

- ¼ cup baby spinach, blanched
- 1 cup broccoli florets, blanched
- 1 tsp. minced shallot
- 2 tsps. extra virgin olive oil
- ⅓ cup vegetable or chicken stock
- ¼ tsp. ground white pepper (or substitute black pepper)
- 1 tsp. finely grated ginger
- ½ Thai chili, seeded and minced
- 1 tsp. finely chopped cilantro
- ½ tsp. lime zest
- 2 tsps. lime juice
- 1 tsp. chopped fresh mint
- 4 oz. salmon or halibut, cut into ½" dice

Combine the spinach, broccoli, ½ tsp. shallot, 1 tsp. olive oil and stock in a blender until smooth. Stir in the pepper and set aside.

Combine the remaining ½ tsp. shallot, ginger, chili pepper, cilantro, lime zest, 1 tsp. lime juice and mint in a small bowl. Add the fish and stir to combine. Form the fish into a patty about ½" thick. Wrap in plastic wrap and refrigerate for 30 minutes.

Heat the remaining 1 tsp. olive oil in a small skillet over medium-high heat. Add the fish cake and cook for 3 minutes, until lightly browned. Turn and cook for 2-3 minutes longer, until just cooked through.

Warm the broccoli puree in a small saucepan over medium heat. Spoon the sauce onto a plate. Set the fish on top and drizzle on the remaining 1 tsp. lime juice to serve.

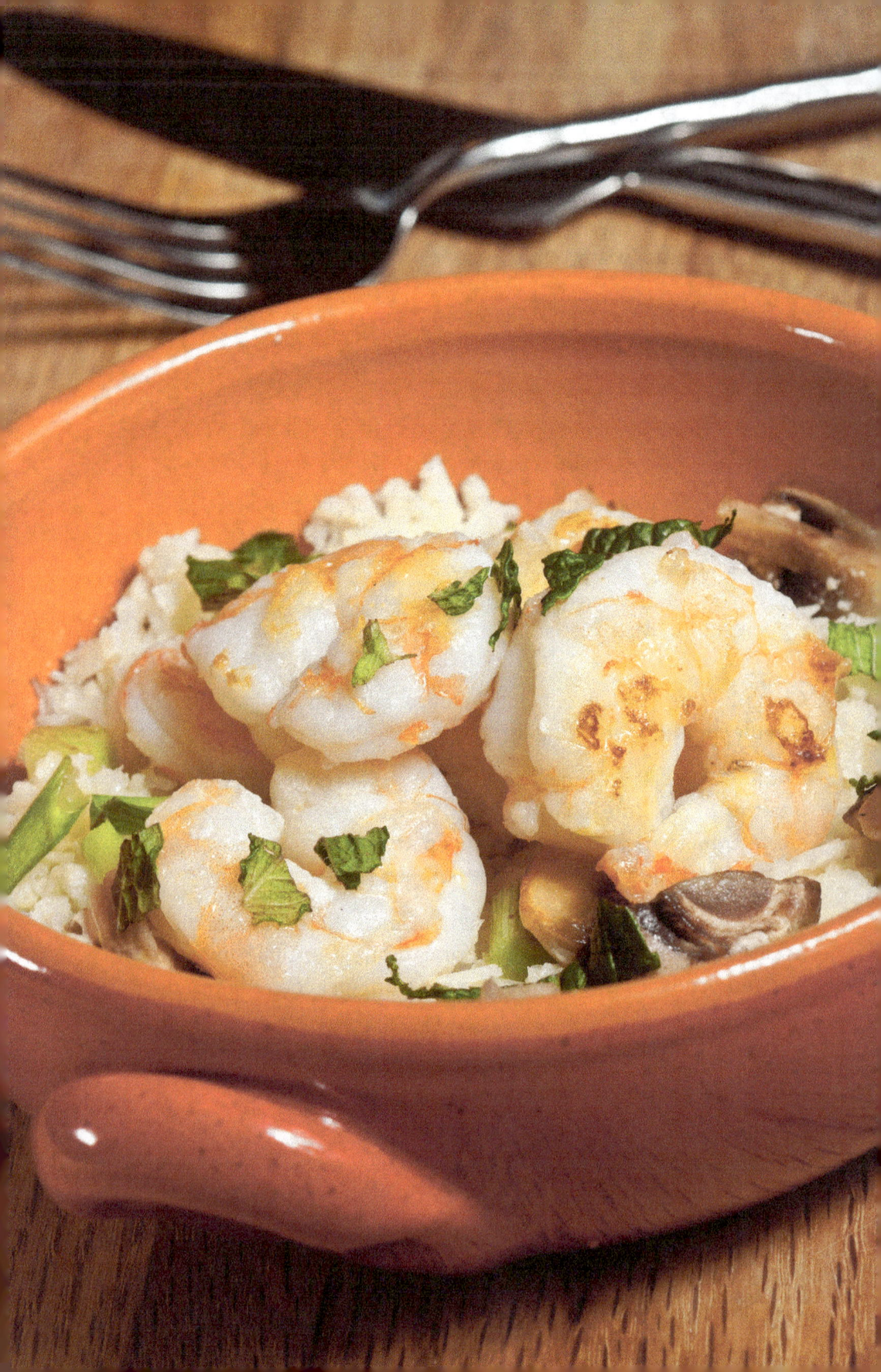

Sesame Shrimp with Orange and Almonds

This Asian-inspired dish is flavored with ginger and orange.

SERVES 1

- 1 cup cauliflower florets, coarsely grated
- 2 tsps. orange juice
- ½ tsp. finely grated ginger
- ¼ tsp. ground coriander
- ½ tsp. minced shallot
- 1 tsp. sesame oil
- 2 tsps. extra virgin olive oil
- ½ tsp. minced garlic
- 7–8 large (31–35 per lb.) shrimp, peeled and deveined
- 1 scallion, trimmed and coarsely chopped
- 4 white mushrooms, quartered
- 1 tsp. toasted sesame seeds
- 1 tsp. chopped fresh mint

Fill a small skillet with water and bring to a boil over medium-high heat. Add the cauliflower and cook for 2 minutes. Drain the cauliflower and submerge it in cool water. Drain and set aside.

Whisk together the orange juice, ginger, coriander, shallot and sesame oil in a small bowl and set aside.

Heat 1 tsp. olive oil in a medium skillet over medium heat. Add the garlic and cook for 30 seconds. Add the shrimp and cook for 2 minutes, until lightly brown on the bottom. Turn and cook for 1–2 minutes longer, until pink and just cooked through. Remove the shrimp from the skillet.

Add the remaining 1 tsp. olive oil to the skillet. Add the scallion and mushrooms and sauté until softened, about 4–5 minutes. Add the cauliflower and stir to heat through, about 1–2 minutes. Remove from the heat and stir in the orange juice mixture. Add the shrimp and toss to coat. Sprinkle on the sesame seeds and mint to serve.

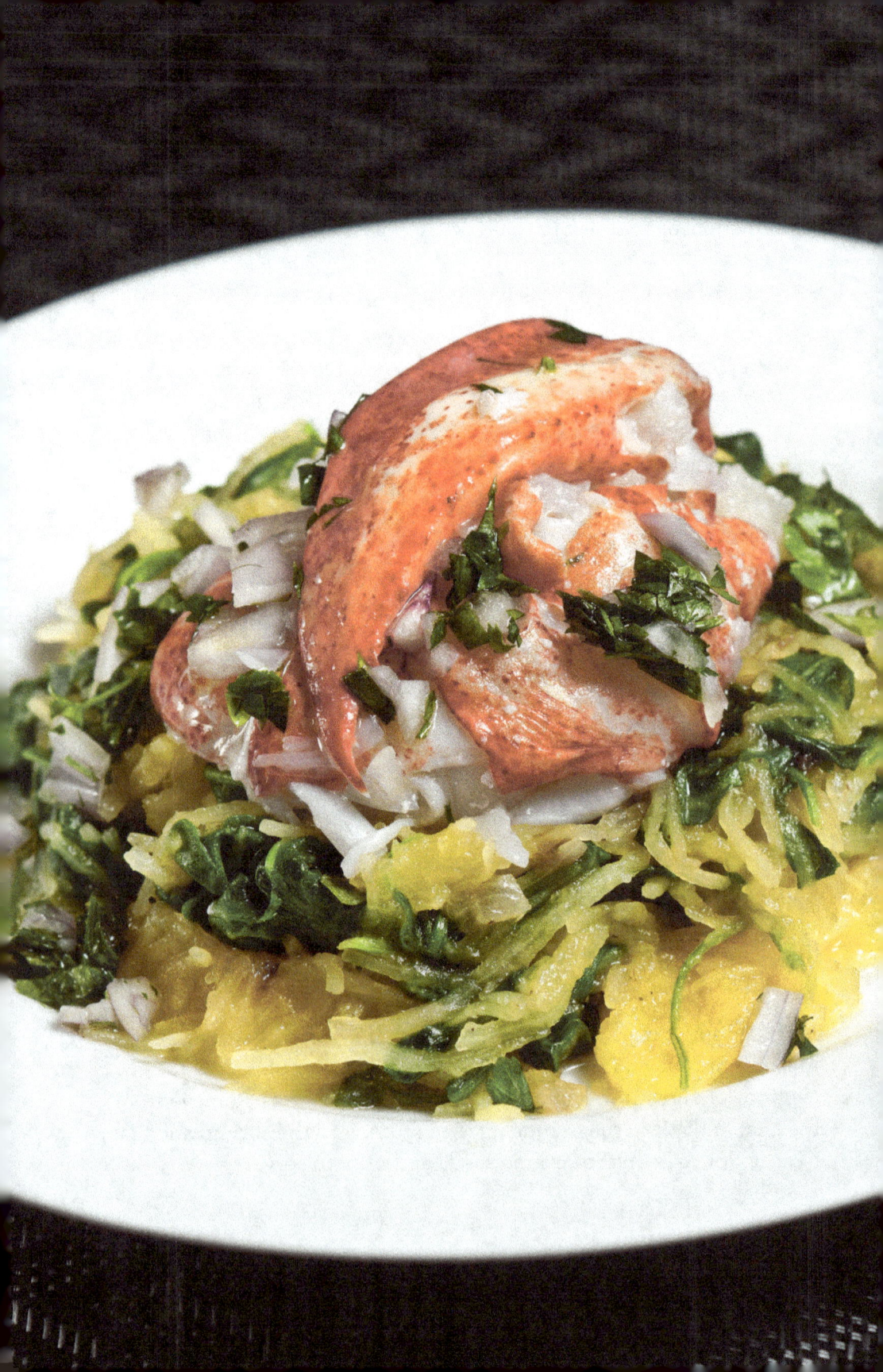

Lobster with Arugula and Spaghetti Squash

If your impression of lobster is "Ugh, too chewy," here is a technique that will change your opinion of it. Undercooking the lobster when steaming it and then finishing it by roasting yields delicious, tender lobster. See the Chef's Tip below for instructions on how to prepare live lobster for this amazing roasted version. Purchase a ½ lb. larger lobster to have extra meat for the breakfast on p. 37 or the salad on p. 83.

SERVES 1

- 3 tsps. extra virgin olive oil
- 1 tsp. minced shallot
- 3 tsps. lemon juice
- 3 tsps. chopped flat-leaf parsley
- 1 (1–1 ¼ lb.) lobster, steamed and meat removed (see Chef's Tip)
- 1 cup arugula (about ½ oz.)
- 1 cup cooked spaghetti squash (see Chef's Tip p. 100)
- ½ tsp. chopped fresh thyme
- ¼ cup chicken stock

Preheat the oven to 400 degrees F. Lightly grease a small baking dish and set aside.

Whisk together 1 tsp. olive oil, ½ tsp. shallot, 1 tsp. lemon juice and 1 tsp. parsley and set aside.

Arrange the lobster meat in the center of the baking dish (you can use a ring mold or simply pile it up, placing the claws on top). Drizzle on 1 tsp. olive oil and 1 tsp. lemon juice. Sprinkle with 1 tsp. parsley. Bake for 8 minutes, until just cooked through.

In the meantime, heat the remaining 1 tsp. olive oil in a medium skillet over medium heat. Add the remaining ½ tsp. shallot and sauté for 1 minute. Add the arugula and stir to coat, about 30 seconds. Stir in the spaghetti squash and thyme, then toss to combine. Add the stock and stir until the liquid is evaporated and the squash is heated through, about 2–3 minutes. Remove from the heat and stir in the parsley and remaining 1 tsp. lemon juice. Season with freshly ground pepper.

Mound the squash and arugula mixture onto a plate. Set the lobster in the center and drizzle on the olive oil/lemon mixture to serve.

Chef's Tip: For tender roasted lobster, you will need to cook the live lobster at home. To cook a lobster, prepare a bowl of ice water large enough to submerge the lobster in (or use a small sink). Bring about 2–3 inches of water to boil in a large stockpot equipped with a steamer rack. Place the lobster into the freezer for 15 minutes, and then use a chef's knife to slice down between the lobster's eyes, or alternately along the entire length of its body. (This cuts through its nervous system, killing it instantly.) Steam the lobster by placing it onto the rack and placing the lid on the pot. Allow the lobster to steam until just red—this should yield slightly undercooked meat. Immediately remove the lobster from the pot and submerge it in the ice water to cool it quickly and make the meat easier to remove from the shell. Remove the claws and tail and discard the rest. To remove the meat, use a mallet or seafood cracker to break into the claws, and kitchen shears or a chef's knife to cut down the center of the tail. Continue cooking the lobster according to the instructions above.

Sea Scallops with Cherry Tomatoes, Avocado and Macadamias

Fresh dry scallops have no added chemicals or preservatives, so it's important to ask for them specifically. Pat the scallops dry before cooking to get a crusty brown sear. The avocado slices may also be briefly pan-fried or grilled for added flavor.

SERVES 1

- 1 tsp. avocado oil
- 1 tsp. chopped flat-leaf parsley
- 6 macadamias, finely chopped
- 2 tsps. extra virgin olive oil
- 4 large dry sea scallops, abductor muscle removed and discarded
- 1 scallion, trimmed and coarsely chopped
- 5 cherry tomatoes, coarsely chopped
- 1 tsp. lemon juice
- 2 tbsps. chicken stock
- ¼ avocado, peeled and thinly sliced

Combine the avocado oil, parsley and macadamias in a small bowl and set aside.

Heat the olive oil in a small skillet over medium-high heat. Add the scallops and cook for 3 minutes, until bottoms are golden brown. Turn the scallops and cook for 1–2 minutes longer, until just seared on the bottom. Remove the scallops to a plate and keep warm.

Add the scallion and cherry tomatoes to the pan and cook for 2 minutes, stirring constantly. Remove the pan from the heat and add the lemon juice and stock, scraping up any bits from the bottom of the pan. Stir in the avocado oil mixture.

Place the avocado slices on the plate with the scallops. Spoon the tomato sauce over top.

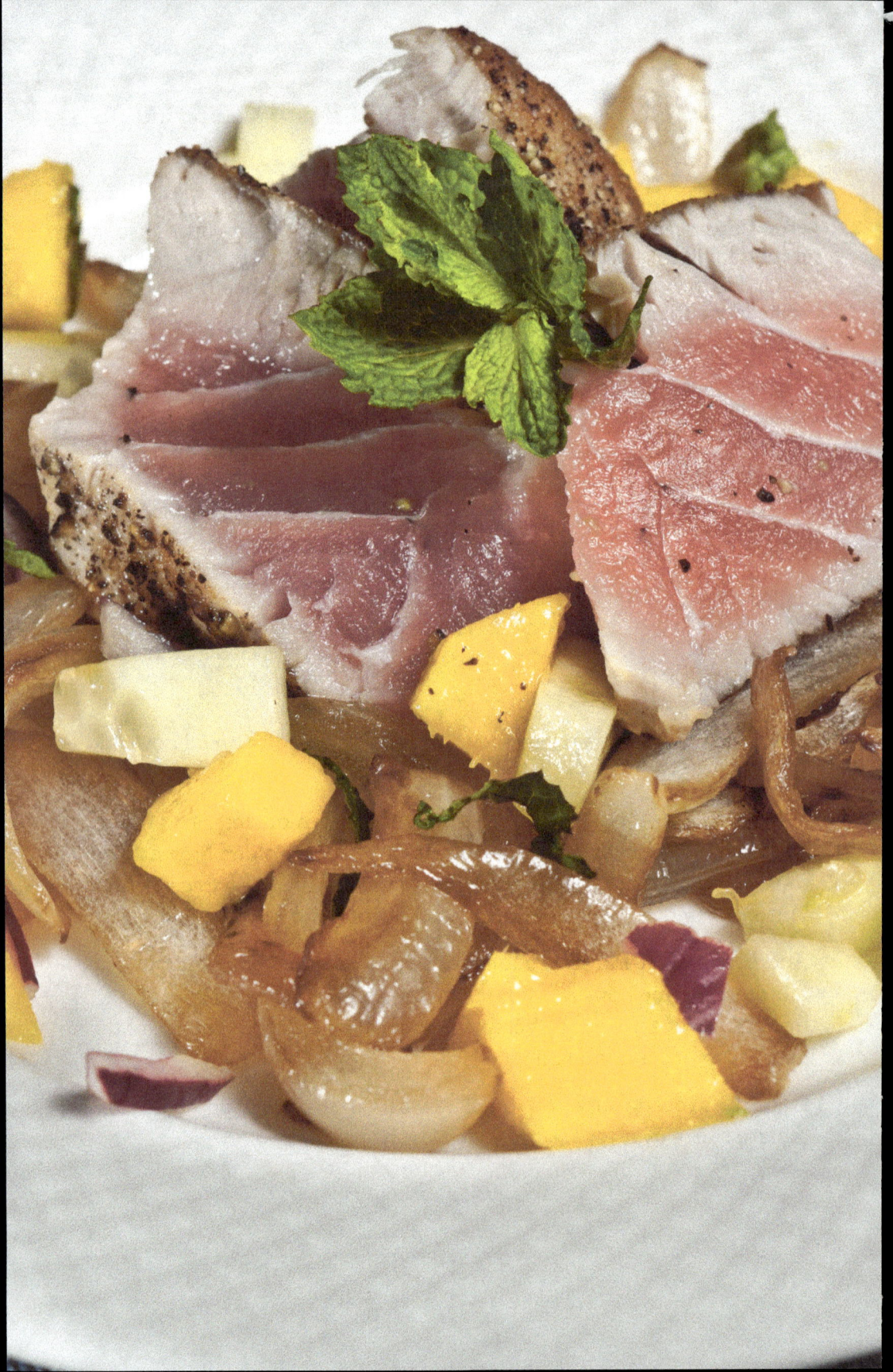

Pan-Seared Tuna with Caramelized Onions and Mango Salsa

This all-purpose tropical salsa is delicious with chicken, steak and pork. Prepare extra tuna for the salad on p. 75.

SERVES 1

- ½ tsp. finely grated ginger
- 1 tbsp. orange juice
- 1 tsp. lime juice
- ½ tsp. crushed red pepper
- 1 tsp. chopped fresh mint
- ¼ ripe mango, peeled, seeded and cut into ½" dice
- ¼ ripe avocado, peeled, seeded and cut into ½" dice
- ¼ medium cucumber, peeled, seeded and cut into ½" dice
- 1 tsp. coconut oil
- 1 tsp. extra virgin olive oil
- ¼ cup caramelized onions (see Chef's Tip p. 56)
- 1 (4–6 oz.) tuna steak, ¾–1" thick

Whisk together the ginger, orange juice, lime juice, crushed red pepper and mint in a medium bowl. Add the mango, avocado and cucumber and toss to coat. Allow the mixture to marinate at room temperature.

Heat the olive oil in a small skillet over medium-high heat. Season the tuna with freshly ground pepper. Sear the tuna for 1 ½–2 minutes until bottom is browned. Turn and cook for 1–1 ½ minutes longer for rare or until desired degree of doneness.

Remove the tuna and add the onions to the pan, stirring until just heated through. Spoon the warm onions onto a plate and set the tuna on top. Spoon on the salsa to serve.

Moroccan Fish Stew

The bold flavor of Moroccan spices blends with tomatoes and fennel in this savory fish stew. Substitute other firm white fish filet like snapper or grouper if halibut is unavailable.

SERVES 1

- 1 tsp. coconut oil
- ¼ sweet onion, thinly sliced
- ¼ fennel bulb, trimmed and thinly sliced
- 1 tsp. grated fresh ginger
- 2 tsps. Moroccan spice blend (see recipe p. 161)
- ¾ cup fish or chicken stock
- 2 plum tomatoes, seeded and coarsely chopped
- 1 (4–6 oz.) halibut or other firm white fish filet
- 1 tbsp. almond slivers
- 1 tsp. chopped flat-leaf parsley

Heat the coconut oil in a medium skillet over medium heat. Add the onion and fennel and sauté until onion is softened, about 3-4 minutes. Stir in the ginger and Moroccan spice blend. Add the stock and tomatoes and bring to a boil. Lower the heat, cover and simmer for 10 minutes.

Season the fish with freshly ground black pepper. Make an indent in the mixture for the fish, place it in the center and recover the skillet. Simmer for 3-5 minutes, until fish is just cooked through. Sprinkle on the almonds and parsley to serve.

Trout with Carrot and Walnuts

This delicious stuffed trout is easy to assemble and baked in the oven. It may also be prepared on the grill.

SERVES 1

- 3 tsps. extra virgin olive oil
- 1 medium carrot, julienned
- 3 tbsps. chopped flat-leaf parsley
- ¼ tsp. chopped fresh rosemary
- ½ tsp. minced garlic
- 1 tbsp. ground walnuts
- 1 ½ tsps. lemon juice
- ½ tsp. finely grated lemon zest
- 1 trout, about 6–8 oz., cleaned

Preheat the oven to 400 degrees F. Lightly grease a rimmed baking sheet and set aside.

Heat 2 tsps. olive oil in a small skillet over medium-high heat. Add the carrot and sauté until just softened, about 1-2 minutes. Remove from the heat and stir in the parsley, rosemary, garlic, walnuts, ½ tsp. lemon juice and zest. Season with freshly ground pepper. Spoon the filling into the trout. Place the fish onto the baking sheet and drizzle it with the remaining 1 tsp. of olive oil. Cover with foil.

Bake the trout for 20 minutes. Remove the foil and bake for 5-10 minutes longer, until the fish flakes easily and is cooked through. Sprinkle remaining ½ tsp. lemon juice onto the filling to serve.

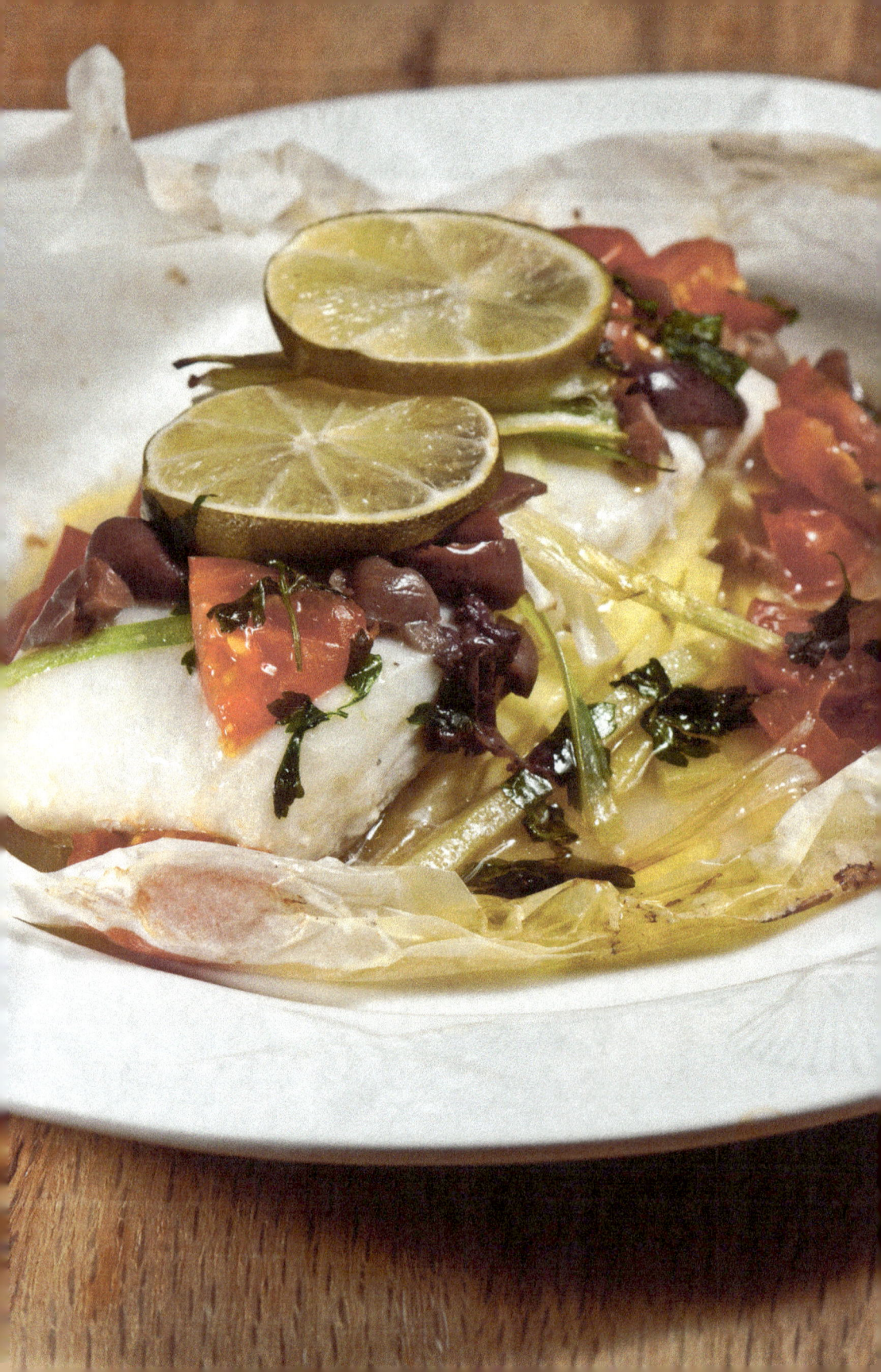

Mediterranean Halibut in Parchment

Cooking in parchment (also referred to as "en papilotte" in French) delivers moist fish with intense flavor in an elegant presentation. The bonus is that it's very simple to assemble and bake. Although slightly less elegant, foil may be substituted for the parchment paper.

SERVES 1

- ½ small zucchini, julienned
- 1 ½ tbsps. extra virgin olive oil
- 1 (4–6 oz.) halibut filet, about ¾–1" thick
- 1 tsp. lime juice
- 6 pitted black olives, coarsely chopped
- 1 scallion, trimmed and julienned
- 4 cherry tomatoes, seeded and coarsely chopped
- 1–2 sprigs fresh thyme
- 2 thin slices lime

Preheat the oven to 375 degrees F. Fold a 15" x 24" sheet of parchment in half. Cut the folded sheet in the shape of a half heart and set it on a baking sheet.

In a small bowl, toss the zucchini with ½ tbsp. olive oil. Unfold the parchment and arrange the mixture on one half, leaving room around the edges to seal the paper. Season the halibut filet with pepper and set it on top. Sprinkle on the lime juice, olives, scallion and tomatoes. Drizzle on the remaining olive oil. Place the thyme sprigs and lime slices on the filet. Fold the other half of the parchment over and line up the edges. Start at the top, folding over about ½" of the edge to seal it. Continue working your way around the edge of the packet, making overlapping pleats until completely sealed.

Bake the fish for 15 minutes, rotating the baking sheet halfway through. Place the packet on a plate and carefully cut open the parchment to serve.

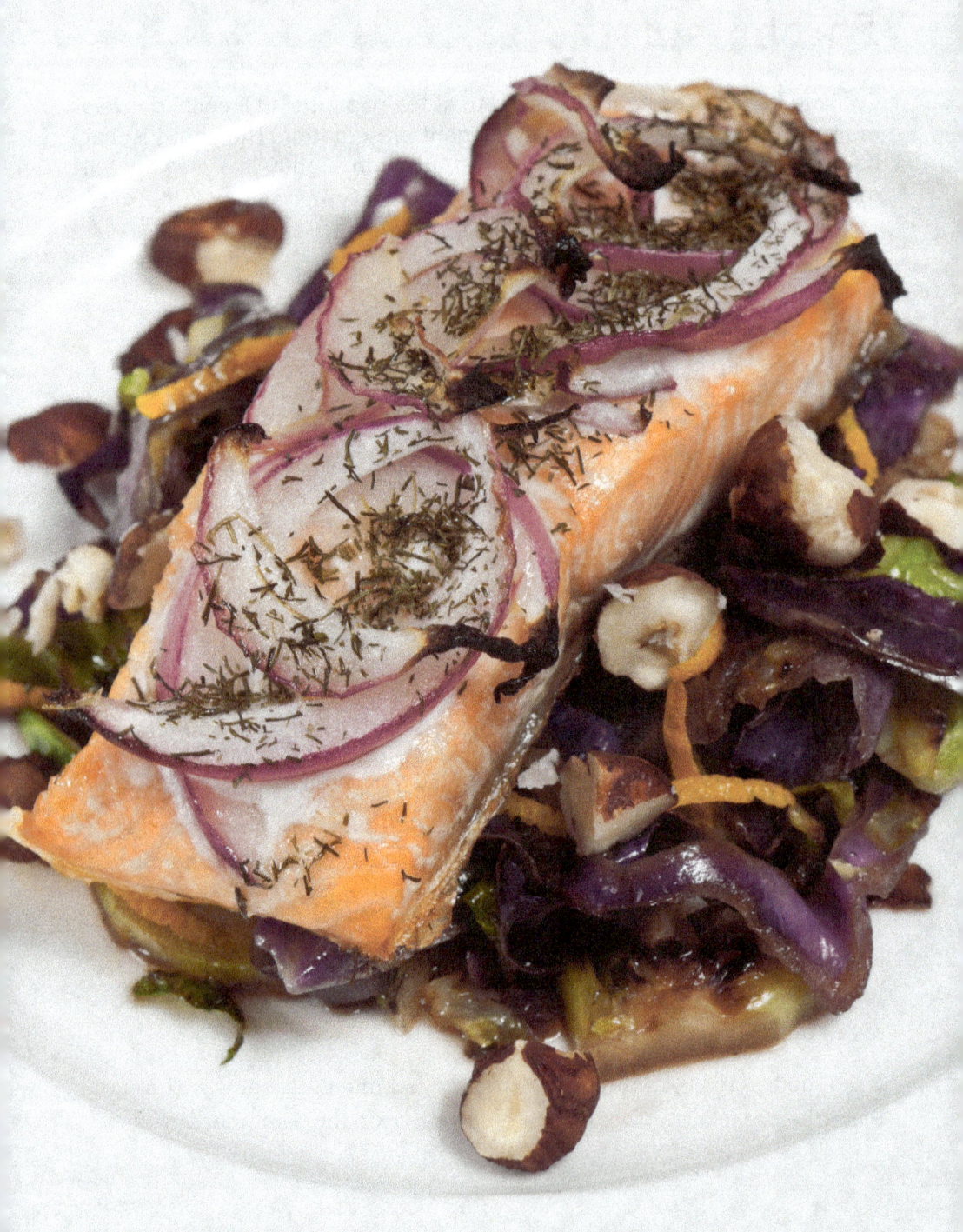

Salmon with Red Cabbage, Brussels Sprouts and Hazelnuts

Roasted salmon is served over a slightly crisp hash of cabbage and Brussels sprouts. Prepare extra salmon for the breakfast on p. 41 and the lunch on p. 87.

SERVES 1

- 1 (4–6 oz.) salmon filet
- 3 tsps. extra virgin olive oil
- 1 tsp. lemon juice
- ⅛ red onion, thinly sliced
- ¼ tsp. dried dill
- 1 cup red cabbage, thinly sliced (about ¼ head)
- 2 Brussels sprouts, thinly sliced
- ¼ tsp. minced garlic
- ¼ cup orange juice
- ½ tsp. grated orange zest
- 1 tsp. lime juice
- 1 tbsp. coarsely chopped hazelnuts

Preheat the oven to 425 degrees F. Lightly grease a rimmed baking sheet.

Place the salmon filet on the baking sheet and season it with freshly ground pepper. Whisk together 1 tsp. olive oil and lemon juice in a small bowl. Stir in the onion and dill. Spoon the mixture over the salmon. Roast the salmon for 10–12 minutes, until just cooked through or until desired degree of doneness.

In the meantime, heat the remaining 2 tsps. olive oil in a medium skillet over medium heat. Add the cabbage and Brussels sprouts and stir to coat with oil. Cook until softened and slightly browned, about 4–5 minutes. Stir in the garlic and cook for 30 seconds. Pour in the orange juice and simmer until the vegetables are just tender and the liquid has evaporated, about 4–5 minutes longer (if you like the vegetables softer, add a little water or stock and continue cooking until the desired texture is achieved). Remove from the heat and stir in the orange zest and lime juice.

Spoon the cabbage mixture onto a plate and top with the salmon. Sprinkle on the hazelnuts to serve.

Pan-Roasted Mussels with Onions and Basil

Pan roasting adds rich flavor to the mussels.

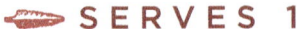 **SERVES 1**

- 2 tbsps. extra virgin olive oil
- ½ tsp. minced shallot
- ½ medium carrot, peeled and finely diced
- ½ leek, white parts only, finely chopped
- ½ celery stalk, finely diced
- 1 tsp. fresh chopped thyme
- 1 bay leaf
- 1 cup seafood or chicken stock
- ½ lb. mussels, scrubbed
- ¼ onion, thinly sliced
- 3 fresh basil leaves, cut into chiffonade
- 1 tsp. lemon juice

Heat 1 tbsp. olive oil in a medium saucepan over medium-high heat. Add the shallot, carrot, leek and celery stalk and cook for 2 minutes. Stir in the thyme and bay leaf. Add the stock and ¼ cup water and bring to a boil. Lower the heat and simmer until vegetables are tender, about 8–10 minutes. Remove and discard the bay leaf. Keep warm.

In a separate large saucepan or cast-iron Dutch oven, heat the remaining 1 tbsp. olive oil over medium-high heat. Add the mussels, onion and basil. Stir constantly for 1 minute. Cover and cook until the mussels are open and the onions are softened, about 3–4 minutes. Remove from the heat and discard any unopened mussels.

Pour the warm vegetable broth into a bowl and spoon in the mussels and onions. Season with freshly ground black pepper to serve.

Red Snapper with Leeks and Saffron

Lightly caramelized roasted leeks are served with marinated red snapper and finished with a saffron-scented sauce.

SERVES 1

- 2 medium leeks, white parts only, sliced in half lengthwise
- 1 ½ tbsps. extra virgin olive oil
- ¼ tsp. dried thyme
- 2 tbsps. lemon juice
- 1 (4–6 oz.) red snapper filet
- 1 carrot, peeled, trimmed and finely chopped
- ¼ cup finely chopped onion
- Pinch of saffron
- ½ cup fish or chicken stock
- 1 tsp. coconut oil

Preheat the oven to 400 degrees F.

Place the leeks in a single layer in a baking dish. Drizzle with ½ tbsp. olive oil and season with pepper. Bake the leeks for 20–25 minutes, until tender and edges are golden brown.

In the meantime, whisk together ½ tbsp. olive oil, thyme and 1 tbsp. lemon juice in a shallow bowl. Add the fish and turn to coat. Allow the fish to marinate in the mixture for 20 minutes.

While the fish is marinating, heat the remaining ½ tbsp. olive oil in a small saucepan over medium heat. Add the carrot, onion and saffron and cook until the vegetables release some liquid, about 4–5 minutes. Add the stock and bring to a simmer. Cook until the vegetables are softened and cooked through, about 4–5 minutes longer. Remove from the heat and stir in the remaining ½ tbsp. lemon juice. Strain the mixture through a fine sieve set over a bowl. Press the mixture with the back of a spoon and scrape any mixture off the bottom of the sieve into the bowl. Discard any remaining vegetables and keep the sauce warm.

Heat the coconut oil in a medium skillet over medium-high heat. Drain and discard any excess marinade off of the fish and pat dry. Add the fish to the skillet and cook, turning once, until lightly browned and just cooked through, about 3–4 minutes per side. Arrange the leeks and fish on a plate and drizzle with the sauce to serve.

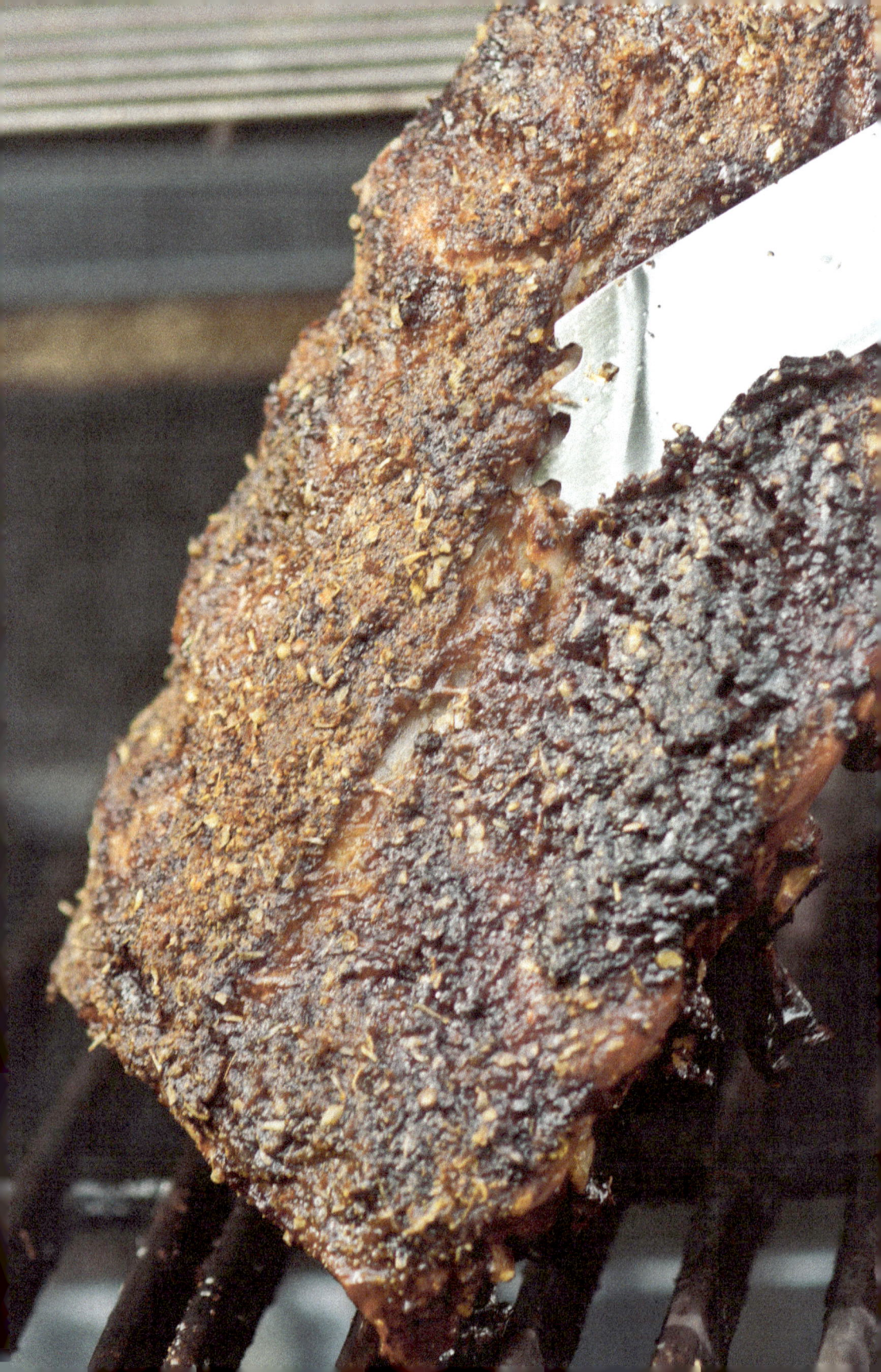

Pork Ribs with Jicama Slaw

This rub combines herbs and spices for robust flavor without adding salt or sugar. The ribs are falling-off-the-bone delicious, whether cooked simply with the rub or lightly brushed with the sauce. Make extra pork to use in salads or for snacks. The rub is also delicious on chicken or steak. The ribs may also be slow-cooked on the grill for added flavor.

SERVES 1

- ¼ tsp. ground cumin
- ¼ tsp. smoked paprika
- ¼ tsp. dried oregano
- ¼ tsp. freshly ground black pepper
- ¼ tsp. chili powder
- 1 tsp. extra virgin olive oil
- ½ lb. baby back ribs
- 1 tbsp. lime juice
- ½ tsp. crushed red pepper
- ½ tsp. chili powder
- 3 tbsps. extra virgin olive oil
- ½ medium jicama, peeled and julienned (about 1 cup)
- 1 medium carrot, peeled and julienned (about ½ cup)
- ½ cup shredded Napa cabbage
- ⅛ red onion, peeled and thinly sliced
- 1 tsp. cilantro, chopped
- 2 tbsps. barbecue sauce (optional—see recipe on p. 164)

Preheat the oven to 300 degrees F. Line a baking sheet with foil and set aside.

Mix the cumin, paprika, oregano, black pepper and chili powder together in a small bowl. Rub the olive oil all over the ribs. Evenly work the rub all over the ribs. Place the ribs meat side up on the baking sheet.

Bake until tender and juicy on the inside and crispy on the outside, about 2 hours.

In the meantime, make the slaw. In a large mixing bowl whisk together the lime juice, crushed pepper, chili powder and extra virgin olive oil. Add the jicama, carrots, cabbage, onion and cilantro and toss to coat.

Remove the ribs from the oven. If using the sauce, place the rack 3–4 inches from the broiler and preheat it. Brush the ribs with the sauce and broil for 2–3 minutes, until the sauce is just bubbly. Serve with the slaw.

Pork Loin Chop with Peaches, Squash and Pecans

This moist pork dish is an easy-to-prepare dinner that's loaded with flavor.

SERVES 1

- 1 (4–6 oz.) boneless center cut pork chop
- 1 ½ tbsps. extra virgin olive oil
- 2 tbsps. coarsely ground pecans
- 1 medium peach, peeled, pitted and thinly sliced
- ½ yellow squash, trimmed and cut into ½" dice
- Pinch ground allspice
- ½ tsp. chopped fresh thyme
- ⅓ cup chicken stock
- ½ tsp. lemon juice

Season the pork chop with freshly ground pepper. Place the pork chop between layers of plastic wrap or in a Ziploc bag and pound out until about ¼" thick. Lightly brush the pork chop with ½ tbsp. olive oil. Place the pecans on a plate and dredge the pork chop in them to evenly coat both sides.

Heat the remaining 1 tbsp. olive oil in a medium skillet over medium heat. Add the pork chop and cook for 3-4 minutes, until lightly browned. Turn the pork chop, lower the heat and cover. Cook for 3-4 minutes longer, until just cooked through. Remove the pork chop from the pan, place on a plate and cover loosely with foil to rest.

Add the peach slices, squash, allspice and thyme to the skillet and stir for 1 minute. Pour in the chicken stock, scraping up any bits and pecans off the bottom. Cook until the sauce is reduced and slightly thickened, about 3-4 minutes. Remove from the heat and stir in the lemon juice.

Spoon the squash and peaches onto a plate and set the pork on top. Pour any remaining sauce over the pork chop to serve.

Pork Tenderloin with Cherries and Kale

The sweetness of sautéed fresh cherries balances the slight bitterness of kale in this easy-to-prepare meal. Make an extra piece of pork tenderloin to enjoy at breakfast (it's delicious in the Pork and Mango Omelet on p. 43) or for lunch paired with watermelon, cucumber and red onion on p. 91.

SERVES 1

- 4–6 oz. pork tenderloin
- 1 tbsp. extra virgin olive oil
- 1–1 ½ cups kale, thick stems removed and cut into thin strips
- 1 tbsp. chopped onion
- 1 tbsp. orange juice
- ½ tsp. finely grated orange zest
- ½ cup fresh cherries (about 2–3 oz.), pitted and chopped
- ¼ cup chicken stock
- ¼ tsp. chopped fresh rosemary

Preheat the oven to 425 degrees F. Lightly grease a baking dish and set aside.

Season the pork with freshly ground pepper. Heat ½ tbsp. olive oil in a small skillet over medium heat. Add the pork and brown it on all sides, about 5-6 minutes. Place the pork into the baking dish and bake for 10–12 minutes, until just cooked through (internal temperature of 145 degrees F). Cover the pork loosely with foil and allow it to rest for 5 minutes.

In the meantime, heat the remaining ½ tbsp. olive oil in the same skillet over medium-high heat. Add the onion and cook until softened, about 4–5 minutes. Stir in the orange juice, orange zest and cherries. Pour in the chicken stock, scraping up any bits from the bottom of the pan. Bring the liquid to a boil. Add the kale and simmer for 4–5 minutes, until the kale is wilted and tender. Stir in the rosemary and remove from the heat.

Slice the pork tenderloin into thin pieces and place them on top of the cherry and kale mixture to serve.

Five Spice Chicken with Tangerine and Fennel

Five spices combine with slightly sweet tangerine and crisp sautéed fennel. Substitute mandarin orange if tangerine is unavailable. Make extra chicken to have it ready to prepare the breakfast recipe on p. 63.

SERVES 1

- 3 tsps. coconut oil
- 1 (4–6 oz.) boneless, skinless chicken breast, pounded out evenly to ¼"
- ½ tsp. five spice powder
- 1 tsp. minced shallot
- 1 tsp. finely grated ginger
- ¼ large fennel bulb, trimmed and thinly sliced
- ½ cup chicken stock
- 2 tbsps. tangerine or orange juice
- 1 tsp. finely grated tangerine or orange zest
- 4 tangerine segments, peeled and seeded
- 1 tsp. chopped fresh Thai basil

Preheat the oven to 375 degrees F.

Brush the chicken with 1 tsp. coconut oil and rub the five spice powder onto it. Season with freshly ground pepper. Heat 1 tsp. oil in a small, heatproof skillet over medium-high heat. Add the chicken and cook until lightly browned on the bottom, about 3-4 minutes. Turn the chicken and cook until lightly browned on the other side, about 3-4 minutes longer. Remove the pan from the heat and place in the oven.

Bake for 8-10 minutes, until just cooked through (internal temperature 165 degrees). Remove from the oven and cover the chicken with foil. Allow the chicken to rest for 5 minutes.

In the meantime, add the remaining 1 tsp. oil in a small skillet over medium heat. Add the shallot, ginger and fennel and sauté until fennel is slightly softened, about 4-5 minutes. Add the chicken stock, cover the pan and simmer for 8-10 minutes, until fennel is tender. Remove from the heat and stir in the juice, zest and tangerine segments.

Slice the chicken into thin pieces. Spoon the fennel onto a plate, top with the chicken and sprinkle on the basil to serve.

Green Coconut Curry with Chicken and Cabbage

Shredded cabbage adds an interesting texture and flavor to this Thai-style green curry.

SERVES 1

- 1 scallion, trimmed and coarsely chopped
- 1 Thai chili, seeded and minced
- 1 tsp. finely grated ginger
- ¼ tsp. minced garlic
- 1 tbsp. chopped cilantro
- 1 tsp. lime juice
- 2 tsps. coconut oil
- 1 (4–6 oz.) boneless, skinless chicken breast, cut into chunks
- ¼ small head cabbage, shredded (about 1 cup)
- ½ cup coconut milk (about ⅓ of a 12 oz. can)
- ¼ cup chicken stock

Combine the scallion, chili, ginger, garlic, cilantro and lime juice with a mortar and pestle (or use a food processor) to form a paste and set aside.

Heat the oil in a medium skillet or wok over medium-high heat. Add the chicken and cook until evenly browned, about 4–5 minutes. Add the cabbage and stir to coat. Add the coconut milk and chicken stock and bring to a boil. Stir in the paste. Reduce the heat and simmer for 4–5 minutes longer, until the chicken is just cooked through and the cabbage is tender. Season with freshly ground pepper to serve.

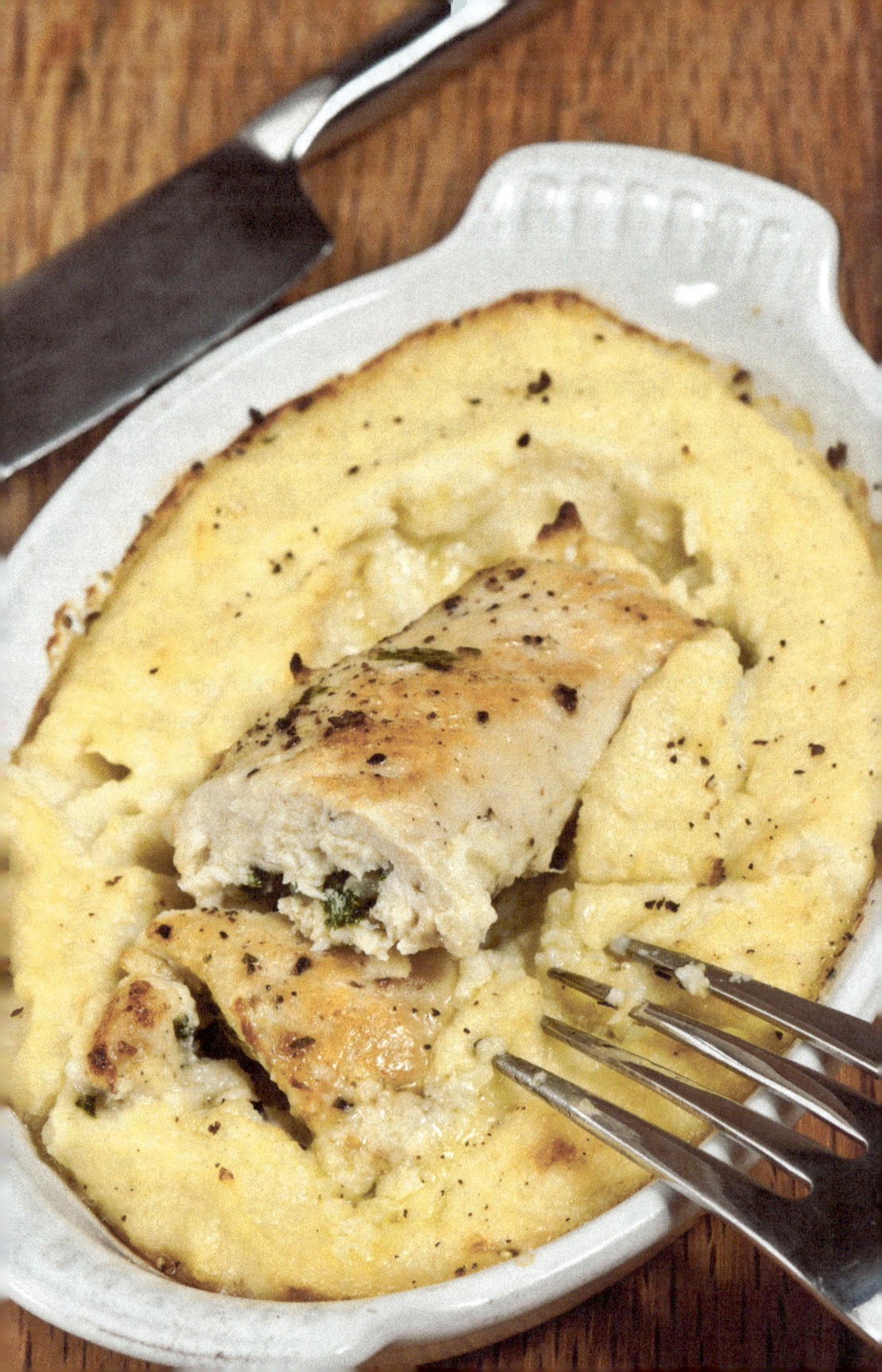

Chicken with Pesto and Cauliflower Puree

Chicken breast stuffed with basil pesto is baked in a creamy cauliflower puree for a delicious, satisfying meal.

SERVES 1

- 3 tsps. extra virgin olive oil
- 2 tbsps. chopped onion
- 1 tsp. chopped shallot
- ½ tsp. chopped garlic
- 1 cup cauliflower florets
- ½ cup chicken stock
- 1 tbsp. coconut milk
- 1 (4–6 oz.) boneless, skinless chicken breast, pounded out evenly to ¼"
- 2 tsps. basil pesto (see recipe p. 165)

Heat 2 tsps. olive oil in small saucepan over medium heat. Add the onion and shallot and cook until softened, about 4–5 minutes. Add the garlic and sauté for 30 seconds. Add the cauliflower, stock and ¼ cup water and cook until the cauliflower is tender, about 8–10 minutes. Remove from the heat and drain off any excess liquid. Stir in the coconut milk. Puree the cauliflower and coconut milk with a blender (or use an immersion blender) and strain it through a fine sieve.

Preheat the oven to 375 degrees F. Lightly grease a small baking dish.

Lay the chicken out on a flat work surface. Spread on the pesto and roll up the chicken, securing it with toothpicks. Heat the remaining 1 tsp. oil in a small skillet over medium-high heat. Add the chicken and brown on all sides, about 2–3 minutes.

Place the chicken into the baking dish. Spoon the cauliflower sauce around the chicken. Bake the chicken and cauliflower for 8–10 minutes, until chicken is just cooked through and the cauliflower is beginning to brown. Allow to cool slightly before serving.

Zucchini-Stuffed Game Hen with Turnip and Mushrooms

Layering grated zucchini between the skin and breast meat yields moist, tender meat. This method works with a roasted chicken as well by simply doubling or tripling the amount of zucchini stuffing. If your hen is on the larger size, you will have some leftover chicken to use in salads or for snacks.

SERVES 1

- 1 game hen, about 1–1 ½ lbs.
- ½ medium zucchini, grated
- 1 scallion, trimmed and coarsely chopped
- 1 tsp. chopped fresh oregano
- ½ tsp. grated lemon zest
- 1 tsp. extra virgin olive oil
- 1 ½ tsps. lemon juice
- 8 medium mushrooms, cut in half
- 1 large turnip, peeled and cut into 1" dice
- 2 tbsps. coconut milk
- ¼ cup chicken stock
- 1 tsp. chopped flat-leaf parsley

Preheat the oven to 400 degrees F.

Remove and discard the gizzards from the inside of the bird's cavity. Rinse the bird and pat dry. Season the hen with freshly ground pepper. Starting at neck, slide two fingers between the meat and skin to loosen the skin. Tie the legs together with kitchen string.

In a small bowl, combine the zucchini, scallion, oregano, lemon zest and olive oil. Carefully fill the space between the skin and meat with the zucchini mixture. Set the bird in a small roasting pan or cast-iron Dutch oven and brush 1 tsp. lemon juice evenly over the skin. Roast for 30 minutes. Add the mushrooms to the pan and stir to coat with juices. Continue roasting for 20–35 minutes longer, depending on the size of the hen (a meat thermometer inserted in thickest part of a thigh should register 170 degrees F).

In the meantime, combine the turnip with the coconut milk and ½ cup water in a medium saucepan. Bring to a boil over medium-high heat, then simmer for 20-25 minutes until tender. Strain the turnip, reserving the cooking liquid. Puree the turnip in a food processor until smooth, adding liquid as necessary.

Spoon the turnip puree onto a plate. Place the hen and mushrooms on top and loosely cover with foil to keep warm.

Heat the roasting pan over medium heat and add the chicken stock to deglaze, scraping up any brown bits. Simmer until mixture is reduced and slightly thickened, about 2-3 minutes. Remove from the heat and stir in the parsley and the remaining ½ tsp. lemon juice. Spoon the juice over the chicken and mushrooms to serve.

Beet and Parsnip Chips with Shredded Chicken

The beet and parsnips chips in this recipe may be made ahead and will stay crisp in a sealed contained for up to 3 days. The beets will shrink to about half their size as they bake. The tandoori-style marinade uses coconut milk and lime juice for acidity instead of the traditional yogurt.

SERVES 1

- 2 tbsps. extra virgin olive oil
- ¼ cup chopped onion
- 1 tsp. minced garlic
- ¼ tsp. ground cumin
- ¼ tsp. ground coriander
- ¼ tsp. ground cardamom
- ¼ ground black pepper
- ¼ tsp. ground cinnamon
- 2 tsps. lime juice
- 2 tbsps. coconut milk
- 2 (4–6 oz.) chicken thighs, skin removed
- ½ medium beet, rinsed and scrubbed
- ½ medium parsnip, peeled
- ½ cucumber, peeled and diced
- 1 tbsp. diced red onion
- ½ plum tomato, seeded and chopped
- 1 tsp. chopped fresh mint or cilantro

Heat ½ tbsp. oil in a small skillet over medium heat. Add the onion, garlic, cumin, coriander, cardamom, pepper and cinnamon and stir well to combine. Lower the heat and sauté until the onion is translucent, about 6–8 minutes. Combine the onion mixture, 1 tsp. lime juice and coconut milk in a blender or food processor until smooth. Cover the chicken with the marinade and refrigerate for at least 10 minutes or up to overnight.

In the meantime, make the chips. Preheat oven to 375 degrees F. Line a baking sheet with parchment and brush with ½ tbsp. olive oil.

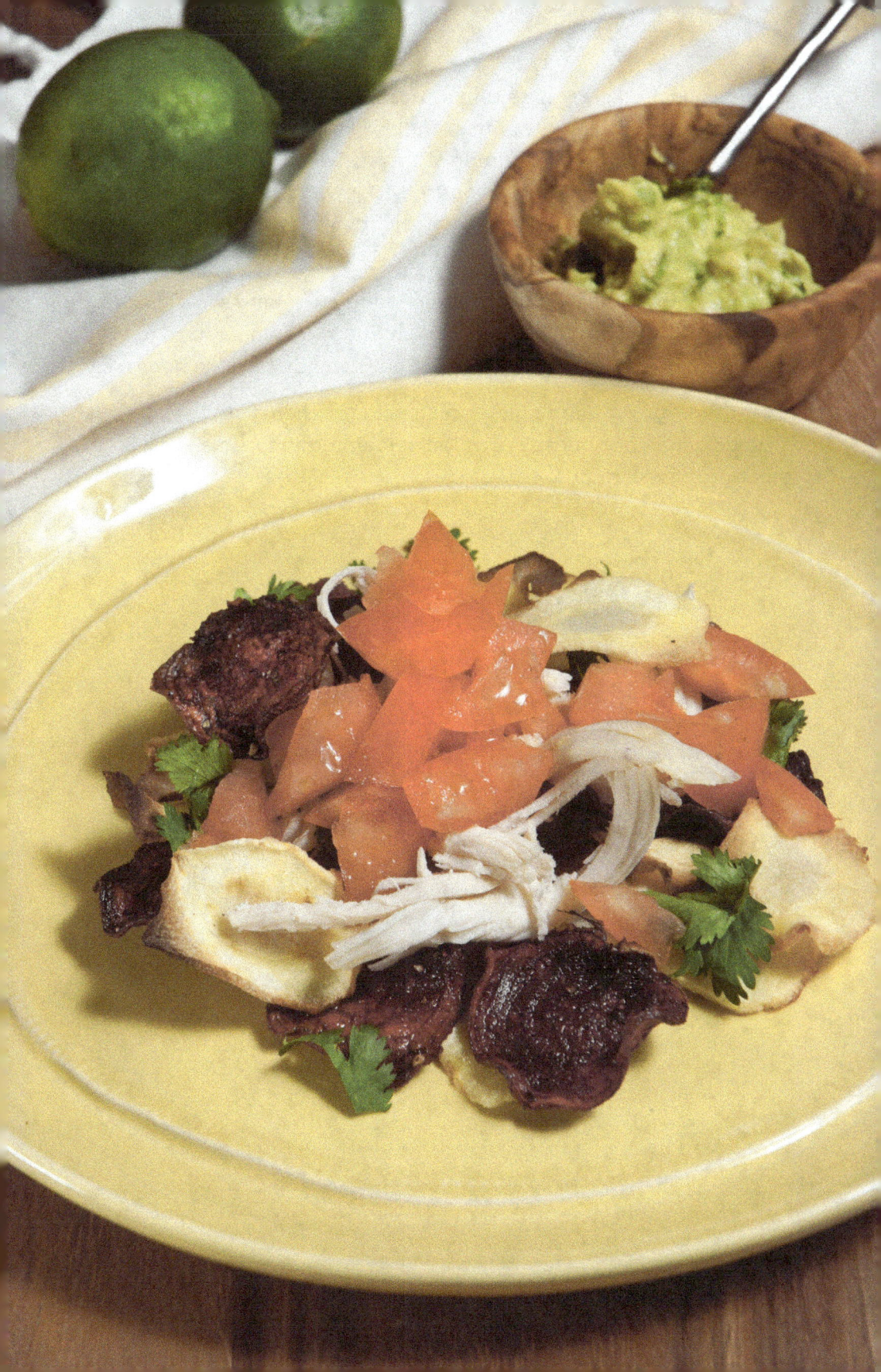

Slice the beet and parsnip as thin as possible with a mandolin or a sharp knife. Lay the slices out in a single layer on the baking sheet. Brush the tops with the remaining ½ tbsp. olive oil and season with pepper. Bake for 15-20 minutes or until crispy and slightly brown. Allow to cool and crisp on a baking rack. If making the chicken right away, leave the oven on.

Place the chicken on a lightly greased foil-lined baking sheet. Bake for 30-35 minutes, until cooked through (internal temperature of 165 degrees F). Shred the chicken off the bones and discard the bones.

Layer the chips overlapping on a plate and top them with the chicken. Sprinkle on the cucumber, red onion, remaining 1 tsp. lime juice, plum tomato and fresh mint to serve.

Turkey, Zucchini and Butternut Squash Strata

Creamy butternut squash is blended with ground turkey and layered with mushrooms and zucchini in this savory casserole. Substitute ground beef or bison for the turkey for a more robust flavor.

SERVES 1

- 2 tsps. extra virgin olive oil
- 2 tbsps. chopped onion
- ¼ tsp. minced garlic
- ¼ cup sliced mushrooms
- ½ tsp. dried oregano
- ½ tsp. freshly ground black pepper
- 4–6 oz. ground turkey
- 1 cup butternut squash puree (see Chef's Tip below)
- ¼ cup chicken stock
- ½ medium red bell pepper, cored and sliced into thin rings (about 6 rings)
- ½ medium zucchini, ends trimmed and thinly sliced lengthwise

Preheat the oven to 350 degrees F. Lightly grease a small baking dish, place it on a baking sheet and set aside.

Heat the olive oil in a small saucepan over medium-high heat. Add the onion and sauté until softened, about 4–5 minutes. Add the garlic and sauté for 30 seconds. Add the mushrooms, oregano and pepper. Cook, stirring constantly, for 1 minute. Reserve half of the mushroom mixture and set aside. Add the turkey to the skillet and cook for 2–3 minutes, until just cooked through. Spoon the mixture into a small bowl. Add the butternut squash puree and chicken stock to the skillet and stir to heat through, about 2–3 minutes. Remove from the heat.

Spoon half of the squash into the bottom of the baking dish. Layer on the turkey. Layer on half the pepper rings and all of the zucchini slices. Spoon on the remaining squash. Spoon the remaining mushrooms and place the pepper rings on top. Cover with foil and bake for 20 minutes.

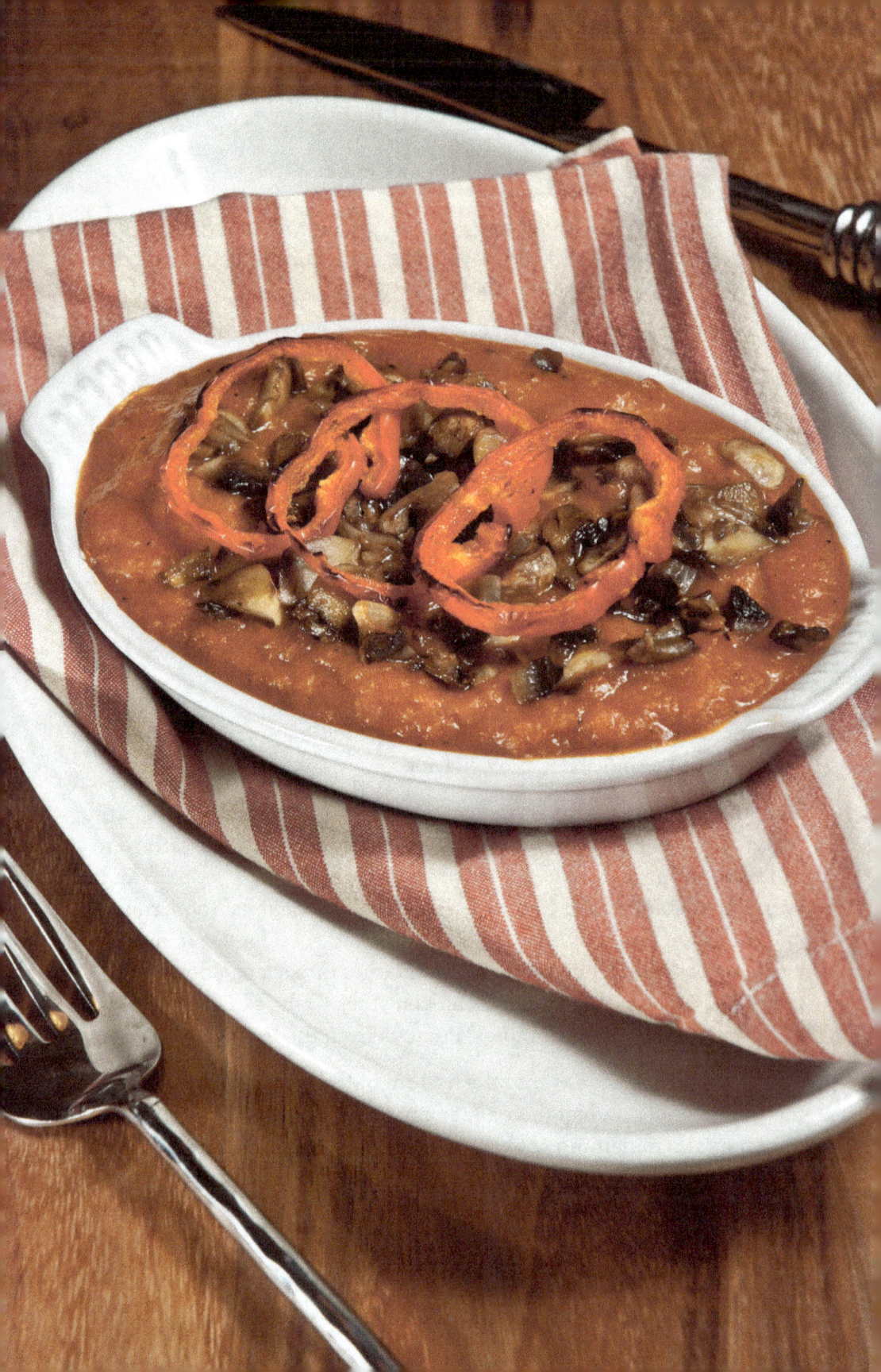

Remove the foil and bake for 15–20 minutes longer, until pepper rings are lightly browned. Allow the strata to cool slightly before serving.

Chef's Tip: To make the squash puree, preheat the oven to 375 degrees F and line a baking sheet with foil. Halve and seed the butternut squash. Place the squash halves, cut side down, on a baking sheet and roast for 35–45 minutes or until fork-tender. Scoop out the flesh and process in a food processor until smooth.

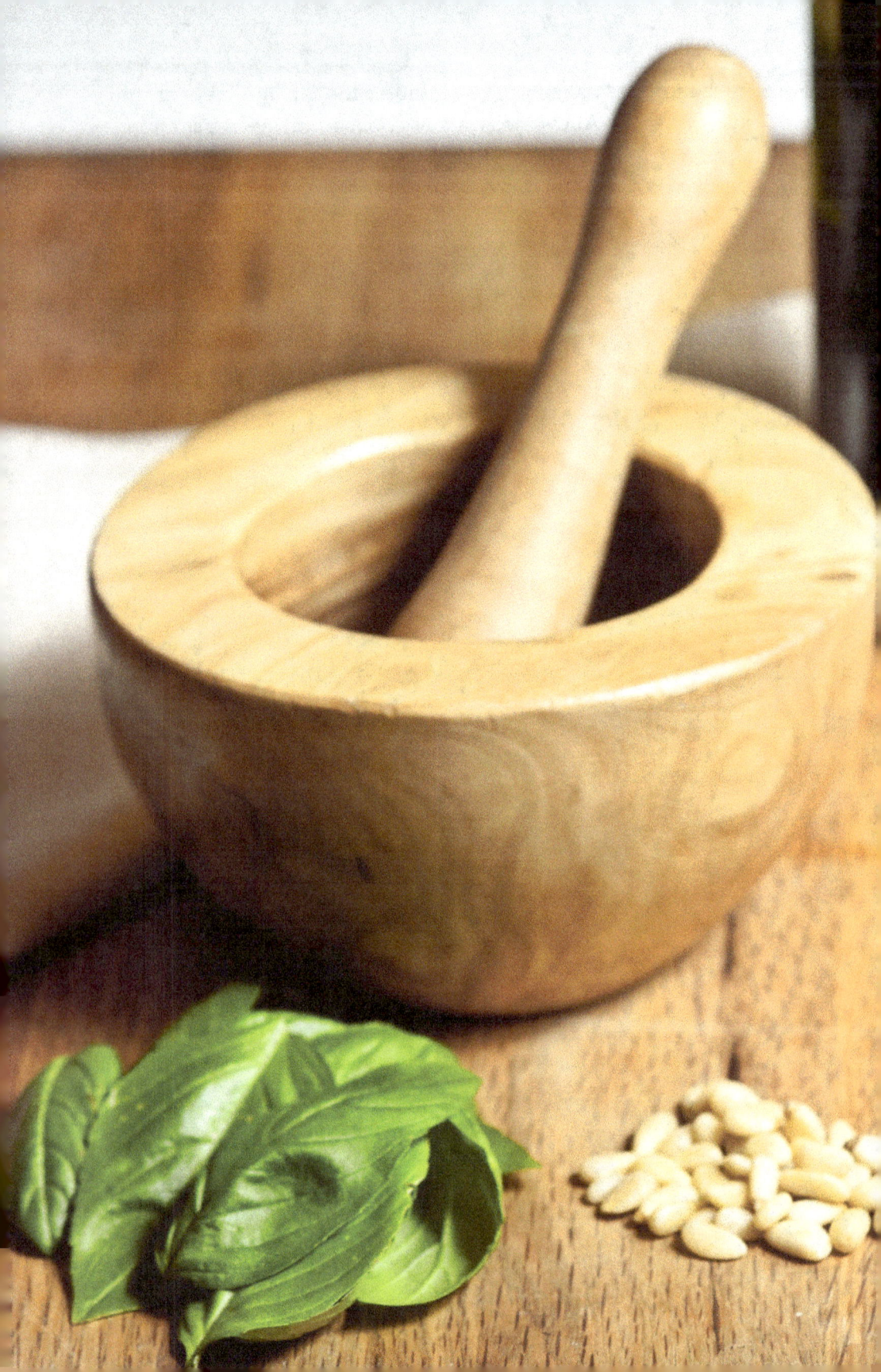

CHAPTER FOUR
Pantry

- Plantain Wraps
- Moroccan Spice Blend
- Chili Powder
- Mayonnaise
- Barbecue Sauce
- Basil Pesto
- Chicken Stock
- Beef Stock
- Fish Stock
- Vegetable Stock
- Sausage
- Pork Belly

Plantain Wraps

These wraps may be used in place of traditional tortillas, especially if you need a little variation from lettuce wraps. They are more flexible than the plantain shells and may be filled and rolled up according to taste. The plantain flour is simply dehydrated, finely ground plantain—no additives or other ingredients—available from specialty stores. It yields an easy-to-roll wrap, similar to a crepe. Unlike recipes using raw plantains, these wraps cook quickly and evenly in a skillet, making them a convenient option.

MAKES 3 WRAPS

- 1 cup plantain flour
- ¼ tsp. baking powder
- ¼ tsp. baking soda
- 2 tbsps. coconut oil, chilled
- 1 scallion, trimmed and finely chopped
- ¼ tsp. cayenne pepper
- 1 tbsp. chopped cilantro (substitute different herbs according to taste)

Combine flour, baking powder and baking soda in a small bowl. Cut the coconut oil into the flour until crumbly. Add 1 cup cold water and mix until just combined. Add additional cold water 1 tbsp. at a time to create a smooth batter, similar to a crepe or very thin pancake batter. Stir in the scallion, cayenne pepper and cilantro.

Heat a small skillet over medium heat and brush the pan with oil. Ladle ⅓ of the batter into the center of the skillet. Immediately swirl the pan quickly so that the batter covers the pan thinly and evenly. Cook for 2 minutes, until the edge just begins to brown and curl. Turn and cook 1 minute longer. Remove from the skillet and cool on a baking rack. Continue until all 3 are complete. Serve within 2–3 hours of cooking.

Moroccan Spice Blend

Making this quick version of the traditional North African spice blend (ras el hanout) ahead of time will simplify preparation of Moroccan-style dishes. It also adds an exotic flavor to ground pork or soft scrambled eggs. It may be made with whole spices, which should be toasted first and then ground.

MAKES ¼ CUP

- 2 tsps. ground nutmeg
- 2 tsps. ground coriander
- 2 tsps. ground cumin
- 2 tsps. ground ginger
- 2 tsps. turmeric
- 2 tsps. cinnamon
- 1 ½ tsps. smoked paprika
- 2 tsps. ground black pepper
- ¾ tsp. cayenne pepper
- 1 tsp. cardamom powder
- 1 tsp. ground allspice
- ½ tsp. ground cloves

Combine all of the spices and store in an airtight container.

Chili Powder

Commercial chili powder often includes salt and sugar, so if a pure version is unavailable, it's best to make your own. It will also ensure that the powder is fresh. Chili powder is easy to prepare and will last when stored in an airtight container for a month.

MAKES ½ CUP

- 1 cup dried chilies (ancho, chipotle, guajillo or mixed), seeds and stems removed

Preheat the oven to 300 degrees F. Line a baking sheet with parchment. Lay the chilies on the sheet in a single layer, and bake for 3-5 minutes until they are dry enough to crumble.

Remove from the oven and cool slightly. Crumble the chilies into a small bowl. Transfer to a spice grinder or food processor and grind to a powder. Store in an airtight container for up to 1 month.

Mayonnaise

This Paleo version of mayonnaise uses olive and coconut oils instead of the soybean oil typically found in commercial mayonnaise. Substitute more olive oil for the coconut for a more robust flavor.

MAKES ⅔ CUP

- 1 egg yolk
- 1 tbsp. lemon juice
- ⅓ cup extra virgin olive oil
- ⅓ cup coconut oil, warmed to a liquid

In a food processor or bowl, combine the egg yolk with the lemon juice and 2 tsps. warm water. With the food processor running (or whisking constantly), slowly drizzle the oil in a thin stream until mixture is smooth and thick. Cover and refrigerate for up to 1 week.

Chef's Tip: If you prefer to not use raw eggs, here is an easy method to pasteurize them:

Place large egg(s) in a saucepan filled with water. Turn on the heat and bring the water up to 140 degrees F, using a digital thermometer for liquids clipped to the side of the pan. Maintain water temperature at 140 degrees F for 3 minutes (and no more than 142 degrees F), adjusting the heat on the burner as necessary. Remove eggs from hot water and submerge in an ice water bath.

Barbecue Sauce

This all-purpose sauce is full of flavor without adding sugar or salt. It's delicious brushed over pork, fish and chicken or as a dipping sauce for shrimp.

MAKES ⅓ CUP

- 1 tbsp. coconut oil
- 3 tbsps. chopped onion
- ½ tsp. minced garlic
- ¼ tsp. dried mustard
- ¼ tsp. chili powder
- ¼ tsp. smoked paprika
- 1 tsp. finely grated ginger
- ¼ jalapeno pepper, minced
- ½ cup fresh pineapple, crushed to release juices
- 2 plum tomatoes, seeded and diced
- ¼ teaspoon ground allspice
- 1 tsp. lime juice

Heat the oil in a small saucepan over medium heat. Add the onion and sauté for 3 minutes. Add the garlic, mustard, chili powder, paprika, ginger and jalapeno and sauté for 30 seconds. Stir in the crushed pineapple with juices, tomatoes, allspice and ⅓ cup water and bring to a boil. Lower the heat to a simmer and cook for 30 minutes, stirring often. Remove from the heat and stir in the lime juice. Puree with a blender (or use an immersion blender) until smooth. Pour the mixture through a fine mesh sieve set over a bowl and discard the solids. Refrigerate for up to 3 days.

Basil Pesto

There are endless variations on pesto—change out the basil for other herbs (mint is delicious with roasted game or lamb), or even substitute spinach, kale or sundried tomatoes. Any nut can be used as well. This Paleo version omits the cheese found in traditional recipes.

MAKES ABOUT 1 ½ CUPS

- 2 cups packed fresh basil leaves
- ½ clove garlic
- ¼ cup toasted pine nuts
- ⅔ cup extra virgin olive oil
- 1 tsp. lemon juice

Combine the basil, garlic, and pine nuts in a food processor and pulse until coarsely chopped. Add the oil and lemon juice and process until fully incorporated and smooth.

Chicken Stock

The key to making a rich chicken stock is to roast the bones before simmering and then simmer for an extended time (anywhere from 8–18 hours). Roasting will remove the fat (which can leave a greasy film) and develop a more complex flavor profile.

MAKES ABOUT 4 QUARTS

- 4 lbs. chicken bones, chopped into 3" to 4" pieces (or use 2 chicken carcasses from roasting)
- 2 medium onions, peeled, trimmed and chopped into 2" pieces (about 2 cups)
- 3 celery stalks, trimmed and chopped into 2" pieces (about 1 cup)
- 2 medium carrots, peeled, trimmed and chopped into 2" pieces (about 1 cup)
- ½ cup white wine (optional)
- 10 black peppercorns
- 2 bay leaves
- 3 sprigs fresh thyme

Preheat oven to 400 degrees F.

Combine chicken bones (or chopped carcasses), onions, celery and carrots in a large roasting pan. Roast until the bones and vegetables are golden brown, about 30–40 minutes.

Pour off any grease and place the pan onto the stovetop over medium-high heat for 1–2 minutes until steaming. Remove the pan from the heat and quickly pour in the white wine (or use water). Return pan to heat. Bring liquid just to a boil and scrape off any brown bits into the liquid. Remove from heat and pour this mixture into a large stockpot. Add the peppercorns and herbs. Add 16 cups of cold water. Bring the liquid up to a boil and reduce to a simmer. Cook for at least 8 hours. Skim off any foam and add water as necessary to keep bones submerged.

Remove from the heat and cool slightly. Strain the liquid through a sieve and discard the bones. Refrigerate until completely chilled through and gel-like in consistency. Skim off any fat that has risen to the surface and reserve for cooking if desired. Refrigerate for up to 1 week or freeze for up to 5 months.

Chef's Tip: Never throw out your roasted chicken carcass. If you don't have time to make stock that day, place it into a Ziploc bag and freeze it until ready to make stock. Allow the carcass to defrost in the refrigerator before using.

Beef Stock

Freezing some stock in ice cube trays (and then storing the cubes in freezer bags) allows for easy portioning.

MAKES ABOUT 4 QUARTS

- 7 lbs. beef bones, sawed into 3" pieces if possible (ask your butcher to do this)
- 2 medium onions, peeled, trimmed and chopped into 2" pieces (about 2 cups)
- 3 celery stalks, trimmed and chopped into 2" pieces (about 1 cup)
- 2 medium carrots, peeled, trimmed and chopped into 2" pieces (about 1 cup)
- ¾ cup red wine (optional)
- 10 peppercorns
- 3 cloves garlic, peeled
- 3 bay leaves
- 2 sprigs fresh thyme

Preheat the oven to 400 degrees F.

Place the bones onto a roasting pan and roast for 1 hour. Remove from the oven. Lay the vegetables over the bones. Return to the oven and roast for 30 more minutes. Pour off any grease and place the pan onto the stovetop over medium-high heat for 1-2 minutes, until steaming. Remove the pan from the heat and quickly pour in the red wine (or use water).

Return pan to heat. Bring liquid just to a boil and scrape off any brown bits into the liquid. Remove from heat and pour this mixture into a large stockpot. Add the peppercorns, garlic and herbs. Add 16 cups of water. Bring the liquid up to a boil and then reduce to a simmer. Cook for at least 8 and up to 18 hours. Skim off any foam and add water as necessary to keep bones submerged.

Remove from the heat and cool slightly. Strain the liquid through a sieve and discard the bones. Refrigerate until completely chilled through and gel-like in consistency. Skim off any fat that has risen to the surface. Refrigerate for up to 1 week or freeze for up to 5 months.

Chef's Tip: Having the beef bones sawed into smaller pieces by your butcher will cut down on the cooking time.

Fish Stock

Fish stocks add flavor to fish and seafood soups and other dishes. This is not a bone broth, in the sense that you don't roast the bones or cook them down (there's no marrow). Unlike chicken or beef, fish stocks are not cooked for more than 25 minutes (or they can become bitter tasting). The vegetables are cut into smaller pieces to accommodate the shorter cooking time.

MAKES 2 QUARTS

- 2 tbsps. extra virgin olive oil
- 1 large leek, trimmed and coarsely chopped (about 1 cup)
- 1 medium onion, peeled, trimmed and chopped into ¼" pieces (about 1 cup))
- 2 medium carrots, peeled and chopped into ¼" pieces (about 1 cup)
- 3 celery stalks, trimmed and chopped into ¼" pieces (about 1 cup)
- ½ bulb fennel, trimmed and chopped into ¼" pieces
- 4 lbs. heads and bones of non-oily white fish, such as sole, flounder, snapper or sea bass
- 1 cup dry white wine (optional)
- 8 whole black peppercorns
- 2 bay leaves
- 6 sprigs fresh thyme

Heat olive oil in a large stockpot over medium heat. Add the leeks, onion, carrots, celery and fennel bulb; cook until vegetables are tender, about 8–10 minutes. Increase heat to medium-high, then add fish heads and bones. Cook, stirring constantly for 5 minutes. Add wine if using. Stir in the peppercorns and herbs. Add 12 cups of cold water. Bring liquid to a boil. Reduce heat to low and simmer 25 minutes, skimming any scum that rises to the surface. Turn off the heat and let cool slightly.

Strain the stock through a fine sieve set over a medium bowl. If you are not going to be using the stock within the hour, chill it as quickly as possible. Prepare an ice bath by filling a large bowl with ice and water. Set the bowl of stock in the ice bath and allow the stock to cool. Cover the stock after it has completely cooled and keep refrigerated for up to 3 days, or freeze for up to 2 months.

Chef's Tip: Ask your fishmonger to save the heads and bones from filets for use in stock.

Vegetable Stock

Roasting the vegetables adds flavor to this rich stock.

MAKES 2 QUARTS

- 2 medium onions, peeled, trimmed and chopped into 2" pieces (about 2 cups)
- 3 celery stalks, trimmed and chopped into 2" pieces (about 1 cup)
- 2 medium carrots, peeled, trimmed and chopped into 2" pieces (about 1 cup)
- 3 garlic cloves, crushed
- 1 leek, trimmed and chopped into 2" pieces (about 1 cup)
- 1 tbsp. extra virgin olive oil
- 1 sprig thyme
- 1 bay leaf
- 6 whole black peppercorns

Preheat oven to 400 degrees F.

In a large bowl, combine the onions, celery, carrots, garlic and leek. Add the oil and toss to coat the vegetables. Arrange the vegetables in a roasting pan in a single layer. Roast for 45–50 minutes, until golden brown and tender.

In a large saucepan or stockpot, combine the roasted vegetables with the thyme, bay leaf, peppercorns and 3 quarts water. Bring to a boil, reduce heat and simmer, stirring occasionally for 1 hour or until the broth is reduced to about 8 cups. Strain the mixture through a fine mesh sieve and discard the solids. Store in the refrigerator for up to 5 days or frozen for up to 2 months.

SAUSAGE

All of the recipes for sausage begin with 8 ounces of ground pork. Simply combine the pork with the seasonings and mix well before cooking.

Andouille Sausage

Andouille sausage is typically smoked, so, if possible, add smoked flavor to this version using a stovetop smoker or smoking gun (available on Amazon or at specialty kitchen stores). Even without the added smoke, this seasoning blend featuring smoked paprika will work well in recipes that call for Andouille. The texture of Andouille is finely ground, so, if possible, ask your butcher to run it through the grinder a second time.

MAKES 8 OZ.

- 8 oz. ground pork
- 1 ½ tsps. chili powder
- 3 tbsps. smoked paprika
- 1 tsp. freshly ground black pepper
- ½ tsp. cayenne pepper
- ½ tsp. ground cumin
- 1 tsp. crushed red pepper
- 2 tsps. minced garlic
- 1 tsp. dried oregano
- 1 tsp. dried thyme

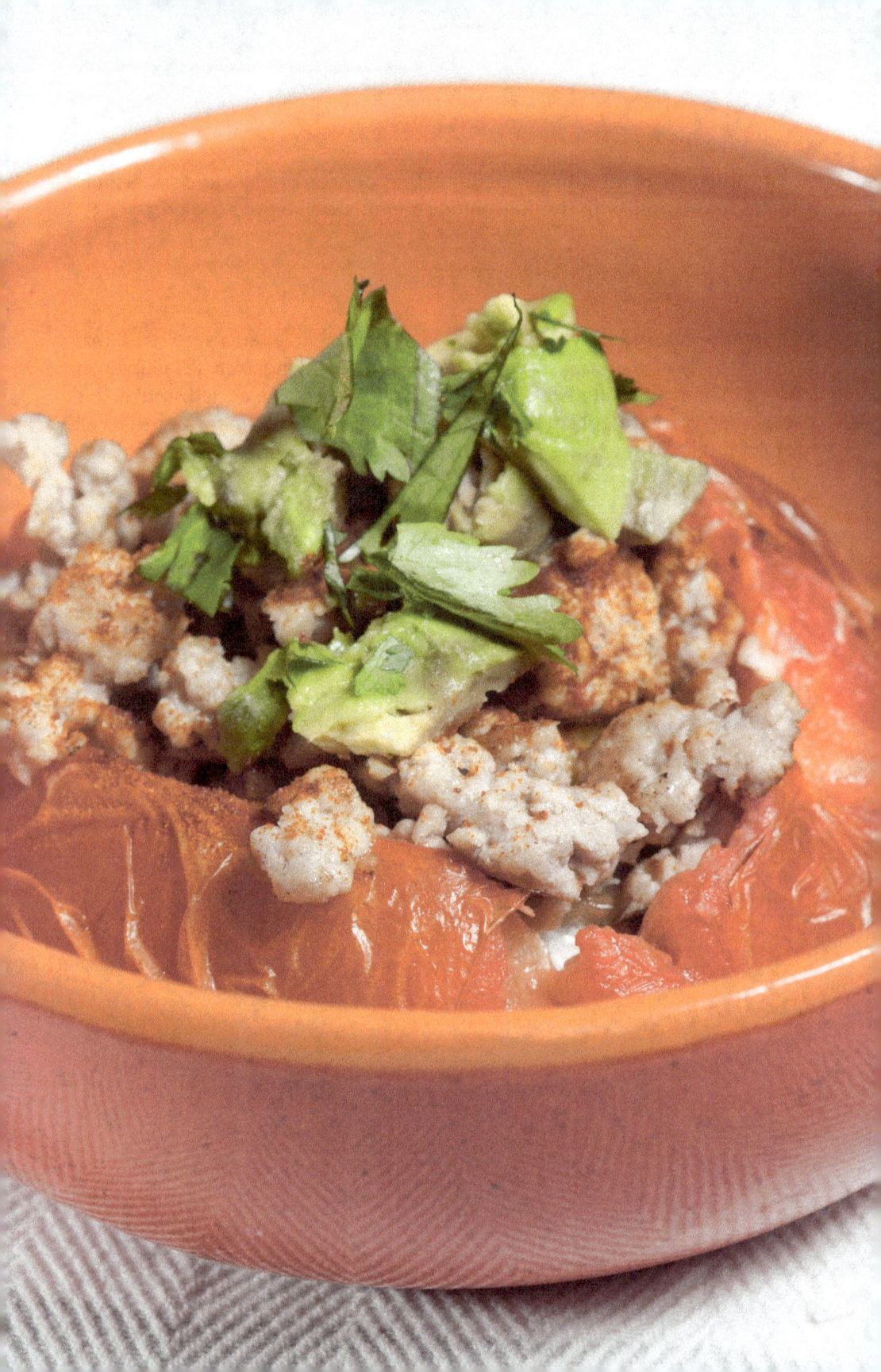

Chorizo

Chorizo may be of either Spanish or Mexican origin, but both types are flavored with smoked paprika. The Spanish version is typically cured (like salami—and not Paleo), so this version is more akin to the Mexican style, as it needs to be cooked.

MAKES 8 OZ.

- 8 oz. ground pork
- 2 tsps. smoked paprika
- 1 tsp. freshly ground black pepper
- ½ tsp. cayenne pepper
- ½ tsp. ground cumin
- 1 tsp. crushed red pepper
- 2 tsps. chili powder
- 2 tsps. dried oregano
- ¼ tsp. ground cloves
- 1 tsp. ground cumin

Italian Sausage

Italian sausage is flavored with fennel or anise and is often sold in two versions: sweet and hot. This blend is somewhere in the middle.

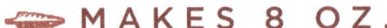 **MAKES 8 OZ.**

- 8 oz. ground pork
- 2 tsps. minced garlic
- 1 tsp. crushed fennel seeds
- 1 tsp. freshly ground black pepper
- ¼ tsp. cayenne pepper
- 1 tsp. crushed red pepper
- ½ tsp. chopped dried sage
- 1 tbsp. chopped flat-leaf parsley

Chef's Tip: Sausage may be refrigerated uncooked for up to 2 days or frozen for up to 2 months.

Pork Belly

Pork belly and bacon come from the same cut of the pig, but pork belly isn't cured or smoked (so it contains no added salt, sugar or preservatives). Spices and black pepper add flavor.

MAKES 1 POUND

- 1 pound pork belly, sliced ⅛" thick
- ¼ tsp. ground cumin
- ¼ tsp. ground coriander
- 1 tsp. smoked paprika
- 1 tsp. coarsely ground black pepper

Heat the oven to 200 degrees F. Line 2 baking sheets with aluminum foil and set the baking racks over top.

Trim away the tough outer rind on the slices of pork belly. Discard the rind. Lay the slices of pork on the racks over the baking sheets. Arrange the slices ½" apart. Combine the cumin, coriander and smoked paprika in a small bowl. Evenly sprinkle the slices with the mixture and rub it into the meat. Bake for 1 hour until cooked through and opaque, but still pliable.

Raise the oven to 400 degrees F. Evenly sprinkle pepper over pork slices. Place pans on 2 oven racks and bake 25 minutes (switching pans between upper and lower racks halfway through the baking), or until pork is golden brown and crisp. Drain the pork on paper towels.

Chef's Note: If you have to buy your pork belly from a butcher, ask them to slice it thinly on their commercial slicer. To slice it at home, freeze the pork belly for 20 minutes, until the edges feel hard and frozen, but the middle is still soft. Use a sharp chef's knife to slice it.

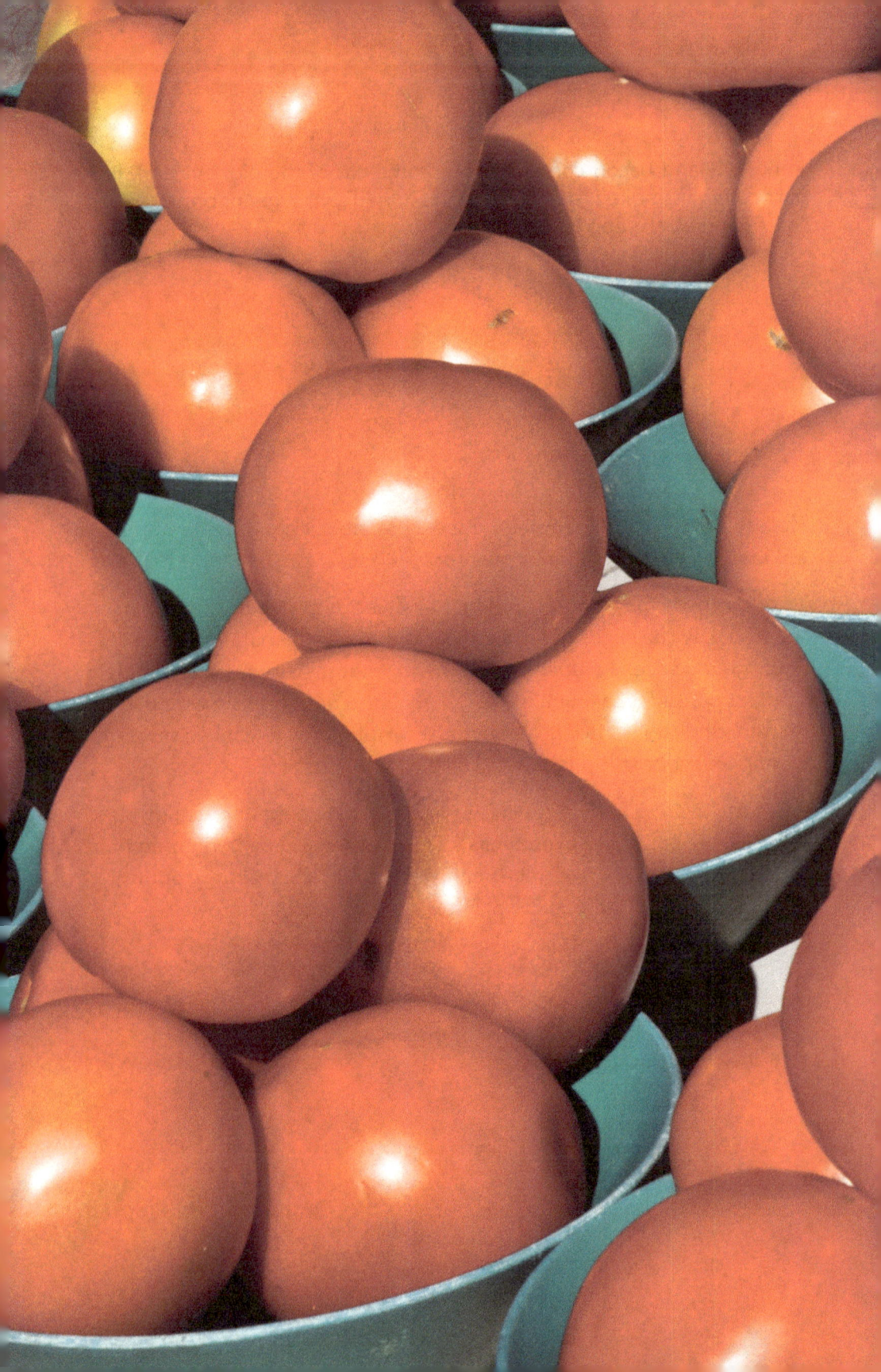

APPENDIX A

PALEO 25 SHOPPING LIST

This list includes pantry basics (like spices) that you may already have, so check what you have on hand before shopping. If you don't have many of the spices on hand, feel free to substitute ones that are readily available and more suitable to your taste, if desired. Some of the pantry items (like Paleo mayonnaise and stocks) may or may not be available to you. If you look for store bought, read the labels to make sure all ingredients are Paleo-friendly. Otherwise, there are simple recipes for them in the Pantry section. The lists are assembled for convenience only, to give you a general idea of what you'll need to purchase if you plan to do all 25 days of meals. The lists contain only what's in the 25 days for breakfast, lunch and dinner, so you will need to purchase extra if you choose to make any of the recipes for pantry items.

Stock Your Pantry

- Avocado oil – 6 oz.
- Beef stock – 1 qt. (store bought or recipe on p. 168)
- Black olives, oil cured (not brined) – 2 oz.
- Chicken stock – 4 qts. (store bought or recipe on p. 166)
- Coconut flakes – unsweetened, 8–10 oz.
- Coconut milk – 2–8 oz. tetrapak or BPA-free cans
- Coconut oil – 1 jar virgin (16–23 oz.)
- Dried Porcini Mushrooms – ⅛ oz.
- Extra virgin olive oil – 16 oz.
- Fish Stock – 1–2 qts. (store bought or recipe on p. 170)
- Garlic – 2 heads
- Ginger – fresh, 4–5" piece
- Lemons – 6–8 medium
- Limes – 6–8 medium
- Paleo mayonnaise – 10–16 oz. (store bought or recipe on p. 163)
- Shallots – 2 ea.
- Tomatoes, sun-dried – 2 oz.

Dried herbs and seasonings: cayenne pepper, bay leaf, black pepper, cayenne pepper, crushed red pepper, dried dill, dry mustard, dried thyme, dried oregano, five spice powder, ground cumin, ground cinnamon, ground cloves, ground turmeric, smoked paprika, star anise and vanilla extract.

Fresh herbs (a small bunch unless indicated otherwise): basil, chives, cilantro (large bunch), dill, flat-leaf parsley (large bunch), kaffir lime leaves, lemongrass (1 stalk), mint, rosemary, sage, tarragon, Thai basil, thyme.

Nuts and seeds (about ½ cup each): walnuts, pecans, sliced/slivered almonds, whole almonds, cashews, hazelnuts, macadamias, pistachios, pumpkin seeds.

Fresh Fruit And Vegetables

- Apples – 4 medium
- Asparagus spears – 10 ea.
- Avocado – 1 medium
- Avocado – 2–3 medium
- Baby spinach – 8–10 oz.
- Bell pepper, red – 1 medium
- Bell pepper, yellow – 1 medium
- Beets – 2 large with greens
- Belgian endive – 1 small head
- Blueberries – ½ pint
- Bok choy – 1 head baby
- Broccoli – 1 small head
- Broccoli Rabe – 1 bunch (about 1 lb.)
- Brussels sprouts – 10 ea.
- Butternut squash – 3 medium (about 4 lbs.)
- Cabbage, green – ¼ head
- Cabbage, Napa – ¼ head
- Cabbage, red – ½ head
- Carrots – 12 (about 1 ½ lbs.)
- Cauliflower – 3 heads (about 7 cups florets)
- Celery – 1 small head
- Celery root – 1 large (about ¾ lb.)
- Cherries – 2–3 oz. (½ cup)
- Cucumber – 5 medium
- Eggplant – 1 large
- Fennel – 1 large bulb
- Frying pepper – 1 small
- Green papaya – 1 medium (or substitute jicama)
- Horseradish root - 1-2" piece
- Jalapeno pepper – 1 ea.
- Jicama – 1 medium
- Kale – 1 small bunch (1 ½ cups trimmed)

- Leek – 4 medium
- Lettuce, romaine – 1 small head
- Lettuce, spring mix – 1 cup
- Mango – 1 medium
- Mushrooms, portobello – 2 caps
- Mushrooms, shitake – 1 lb.
- Mushrooms, white – 3 lbs.
- Mustard greens – 1 small bunch (about ¾ lb.)
- Onions, red – 4–5
- Onions, sweet – 4–6
- Oranges – 2 medium
- Parsnip – 2 medium
- Peach – 1 medium
- Pear – 1 medium
- Pineapple – ¼ cup cubes
- Pumpkin – 1 small pie pumpkin, about 2–2 ½ lb. (substitute butternut squash if unavailable)
- Radish – 2 ea.
- Scallions – 12 ea.
- Sweet potatoes – 3 medium
- Swiss chard – 1 small bunch (1 cup)
- Tangerine – 1 small
- Thai chili peppers – 4 (or substitute 2 jalapenos)
- Tomatoes, cherry – 2–3 pints
- Tomatoes, plum – 17–20 medium
- Tomatoes, slicing – 3 medium
- Turnips – 2 medium
- Watercress – 2 bunches
- Watermelon – 1 cup cubes
- Yellow squash – 1 medium
- Zucchini – 3 medium

Fresh Proteins

- Beef short-ribs (bone-in) – ½ lb.
- Beef tenderloin – 9–10 oz.
- Chicken breast (boneless, skinless) 5 ea. (6–8 oz.)
- Clams, small – ¼ lb.
- Crab meat – 10 oz.
- Eggs – 30–35 ea.
- Game hen – 1 ea. (1–1 ½ lbs.)
- Ground beef – 2 oz.
- Ground pork – 11 oz.
- Ground turkey – 12 oz.
- Ground veal – 2 oz. (substitute beef if unavailable)
- Halibut – 12–16 oz.
- Lamb shoulder chop – 1 ea. (6–8 oz.)
- Lobster, whole – 1 ½–2 lbs.
- Pork, baby back ribs – ½ lb.
- Pork, belly – 2 oz.
- Pork, boneless loin chop – 6 oz.
- Pork tenderloin – 1 ea. (1–1 ½ lbs.)
- Red snapper – 4–6 oz.

- Salmon – 1 ½ lb.
- Shrimp – 1/4 lb. (large, 31–35 per lb.)
- Shrimp, precooked – 2 lbs. (large, 31–35 per lb.)
- Sirloin steak – 4 oz.
- Swiss chard – 1 small bunch
- Trout – 6 oz.
- Tuna filet – 8–10 oz.
- Turkey cutlet – 6 oz.
- Veal, cutlet – 4 oz.
- Veal, rib chop – 8–10 oz.

APPENDIX B

PALEO 25 MENUS

DAY 1

- Italian Fried Eggs with Sausage and Peppers
- Crab, Fennel and Asparagus Salad
- Spicy Lamb Burger with Orange Herb Slaw

DAY 2

- Asparagus, Egg and Tomato Tart
- Shrimp Papaya Salad with Cashews
- Five Spice Chicken with Tangerine and Fennel

DAY 3

- Bok Choy, Carrot and Radish Omelet Soup
- Spicy Chicken Salad with Mustard Greens
- Salmon with Red Cabbage, Brussels Sprouts and Hazelnuts

DAY 4

- Salmon Deviled Eggs
- Pork Tenderloin with Spinach, Orange and Onions
- Red Snapper with Leeks and Saffron

DAY 5

- Portobello, Sausage and Egg Stack
- Roasted Beets with Salmon, Walnuts and Mint
- Meatloaf with Roasted Red Pepper and Cauliflower

DAY 6

- Andouille-Stuffed Tomato
- Shrimp, Red Pepper and Almond Soup
- Pan-Seared Tuna with Caramelized Onions and Mango Salsa

DAY 7

- Pumpkin, Pecan and Coconut Breakfast Bowl
- Tuna Filet with Saffron Slaw
- Lamb Tagine with Star Anise

DAY 8

- Shrimp and Dill Egg Custard
- Roasted Eggplant and Tomato Soup
- Pork Tenderloin with Cherries and Kale

DAY 9

- Scrambled Egg Soup with Spinach
- Watermelon, Cucumber and Red Onion with Pork
- Sea Scallops with Cherry Tomatoes, Avocado and Almonds

DAY 10

- Pork and Mango Omelet
- Veal Scallops with Cherry Tomatoes and Celery
- Chicken with Pesto and Cauliflower Puree

DAY 11

- Sweet Potato Skin with Spinach and Italian Sausage
- Chicken Salad with Carrot, Radish and Cucumber
- Moroccan Fish Stew

DAY 12

- Salmon, Egg and Sweet Potato Pancake
- Celery Root, Leek and Pork Belly Soup
- Veal Chop with Broccoli Rabe

DAY 13

- Blueberry Almond Custard
- Beef Short-Rib and Vegetable Soup
- Mediterranean Halibut in Parchment

DAY 14

- Sweet Potato Hash with Turkey and Egg
- Seafood and Butternut Squash Chowder
- Zucchini-Stuffed Game Hen with Turnip and Mushrooms

DAY 15

- Hard-Cooked Eggs with Crab, Avocado and Belgian Endive
- Turkey with Roasted Sweet Potato, Turnip and Pear
- Pork Loin Chop with Peaches, Squash and Pecans

DAY 16

- Tuna with Poached Egg and Cherry Tomato Salsa
- Curried Zucchini Spinach Soup
- Beet and Parsnip Chips with Shredded Chicken

DAY 17

- Swiss Chard, Pork Belly and Bell Pepper Frittata
- Spicy Sweet Potato and Parsnip Soup
- Chili and Mint Fish Cake with Broccoli Puree

DAY 18

- Turkey, Cauliflower and Apple Soup
- Seafood and Avocado Salad
- Filet Mignon with Celery Root and Mushrooms

DAY 19

- Coddled Egg with Sun-Dried Tomatoes and Mushrooms
- Steak with Mango, Arugula and Pistachios
- Trout with Carrot and Walnuts

DAY 20

- Salmon, Avocado and Pistachio Wraps
- Watercress and Sweet Potato Soup
- Green Coconut Curry with Chicken and Cabbage

DAY 21

- Steak, Pepper and Egg with Arugula Pesto
- Spaghetti Squash Primavera with Chicken
- Sesame Shrimp with Orange and Almonds

DAY 22

- Baked Tomato with Caramelized Onions and Egg
- Chilled Cucumber, Avocado and Shrimp Soup
- Turkey, Zucchini and Butternut Squash Strata

DAY 23

- Five Spice Chicken and Egg Scramble
- Wild Mushroom Soup
- Pork Ribs with Jicama Slaw

DAY 24

- Roasted Eggplant and Cherry Tomatoes with Egg
- Cabbage, Carrot and Apple Slaw with Chicken
- Lobster with Arugula and Spaghetti Squash

DAY 25

- Eggs Lobster Oscar with Asparagus and Cauliflower
- Chicken and Coconut Soup with Cauliflower
- Pan-Roasted Mussels with Onions and Basil

Thank you for purchasing this book. I am pleased to have you along for the journey to better health and better eating. I know you could have picked from dozens of cookbooks about Paleo, so to show my appreciation, I'd like to offer you a bonus: *PALEO 25—TEN TERRIFIC SNACK RECIPES*. Simply sign up on my website www.donnaleahy.com and I will send you the PDF. I will include you on my list for free stuff and also periodically send you any exclusive special offerings. As an experienced chef and author, I write cookbooks on a variety of topics and themes. So even if you find Paleo is not the right eating plan for you, my other cookbooks may interest you as well.

If you have a moment to post a review of this book, I'd really appreciate it. This type of feedback will help me continue to write the kind of cookbooks that you want to use.

Thanks again, I look forward to hearing from you.

Chef Donna

INDEX

Andouille-Stuffed Tomato, 27
Apple
  blueberry almond custard, 53
  cabbage, carrot and apple slaw with chicken, 95
  celery root, leek and pork belly soup, 92
  turkey, cauliflower and apple soup, 65
Asparagus
  asparagus, egg and tomato tart, 49
  crab, fennel and asparagus salad, 84
  eggs lobster Oscar with asparagus and cauliflower, 37
  how to blanch, 38
Asparagus, Egg and Tomato Tart, 49
Avocado
  chilled cucumber, avocado and shrimp soup, 79
  hard-cooked eggs with crab, avocado and Belgian endive, 39
  pan-seared tuna with caramelized onions and mango salsa, 133
  sea scallops with cherry tomatoes, avocado and almonds, 131
  seafood and avocado salad, 83

Baby spinach
  chili and mint fish cake with broccoli puree, 125
  curried zucchini spinach soup, 106
  pork tenderloin with spinach, orange and onions, 89
  scrambled egg soup with spinach, 61
  sweet potato skin with spinach and Italian sausage, 45
Baked Tomato with Caramelized Onions and Egg, 56
Barbecue Sauce, 164
Beef
  beef short rib and vegetable soup,
  beef stock, 168
  filet mignon with celery root and mushrooms, 120
  steak with mango, arugula and peaches, 72
  steak, pepper and egg with arugula pesto, 25
Beef Short-Rib and Vegetable Soup, 73
Beef Stock, 168
Beef tenderloin
  filet mignon with celery root and mushrooms, 120
  steak, pepper and egg with arugula pesto, 25
Beet and Parsnip Chips with Shredded Chicken, 152
Beets
  beet and parsnip chips with shredded chicken, 152
  how to roast, 87
  roasted beets with salmon, walnuts and mint, 87
Belgian endive
  hard-cooked eggs with crab, avocado and Belgian endive, 39

Bell pepper
- how to roast, 82
- shrimp, red pepper and almond soup, 81
- steak, pepper and egg with arugula pesto, 25
- Swiss chard, pork belly and bell pepper frittata, 57
- turkey, zucchini and butternut squash strata, 155

Blueberry Almond Custard, 53

Bok Choy, Carrot and Radish Omelet Soup, 62

Broccoli
- chili and mint fish cake with broccoli puree, 79
- lamb tagine with star anise, 116
- spaghetti squash primavera with chicken, 98

Broccoli rabe
- how to blanch, 123
- veal chop with broccoli rabe, 122

Brussels sprouts
- salmon with red cabbage, Brussels sprouts and hazelnuts, 139

Butternut squash
- how to roast and puree, 157
- seafood and squash chowder, 76
- spicy sweet potato and parsnip soup, 110
- turkey, zucchini and butternut squash strata, 155

Cabbage
- cabbage, carrot and apple slaw with chicken, 95
- green coconut curry with chicken and cabbage, 147
- salmon with red cabbage, Brussels sprouts and hazelnuts, 139

Cabbage, Carrot and Apple Slaw with Chicken, 95

Caramelized onions
- baked tomato with caramelized onions and egg, 56
- how to caramelize onions, 56
- pan-seared tuna with caramelized onions and mango salsa, 133

Carrots
- chicken salad with carrot, radish and cucumber, 97
- pan-roasted mussels with onions and basil, 140
- pork ribs with jicama slaw, 143
- red snapper with leeks and saffron, 141
- spicy lamb burger with orange herb slaw, 115
- trout with carrot and walnuts, 135

Cauliflower
- chicken and coconut soup with cauliflower, 101
- chicken with pesto and cauliflower puree, 149
- eggs lobster Oscar with asparagus and cauliflower, 37
- meatloaf with roasted red pepper and cauliflower, 117
- seafood and squash chowder, 76
- sesame shrimp with orange and almonds, 129

Celery root
- celery root, leek and pork belly soup, 92
- filet mignon with celery root and mushrooms, 120

Celery Root, Leek and Pork Belly Soup, 92

Cherries
- pork tenderloin with cherries and kale, 145

Chicken
- chicken and coconut soup with cauliflower, 101
- chicken salad with carrot, radish and cucumber, 97
- chicken stock, 166
- five spice chicken and egg scramble, 63
- five spice chicken with tangerine and fennel, 146
- green coconut curry with chicken and cabbage, 95
- spaghetti squash primavera with chicken, 98
- spicy chicken salad with mustard greens, 93

Chicken and Coconut Soup with Cauliflower, 101

Chicken Salad with Carrot, Radish and Cucumber, 97

Chicken Stock, 166

Chicken with Pesto and Cauliflower Puree, 149

Chili and Mint Fish Cake with Broccoli Puree, 125

Chili Powder, 162

Chilled Cucumber, Avocado and Shrimp Soup, 79

Clams
- how to steam, 77
- seafood and butternut squash chowder, 76

Coddled Egg with Sun-Dried Tomatoes and Mushrooms, 55

Crab
- crab, fennel and asparagus salad, 84
- hard-cooked eggs with crab, avocado and Belgian endive, 39
- seafood and avocado salad, 83

Crab, Fennel and Asparagus Salad, 84

Cucumber
- chicken salad with carrot, radish and cucumber, 97
- chilled cucumber, avocado and shrimp, 79
- watermelon, cucumber and red onion with pork, 91

Curried Zucchini Spinach Soup, 105

Eggplant
- roasted eggplant and tomato soup, 109
- roasted eggplant with cherry tomatoes and egg, 59

Eggs Lobster Oscar with Asparagus and Cauliflower, 37

Fennel
- crab, fennel and asparagus salad, 84
- fish stock, 170
- five spice chicken with tangerine and fennel, 146
- morrocan fish stew, 134

Filet Mignon with Celery Root and Mushrooms, 120

Fish
- fish stock, 170
- Mediterranean halibut in parchment, 137
- Moroccan fish stew, 134
- red snapper with leeks and saffron, 141
- salmon deviled eggs, 31
- salmon with red cabbage, Brussels sprouts and hazelnuts, 139

salmon, avocado and pistachio wraps, 35
salmon, egg and sweet potato pancake, 31
Fish Stock, 170
Five Spice Chicken and Egg Scramble, 63
Five Spice Chicken with Tangerine and Fennel, 146
Frying pepper
   Italian fried eggs with sausage and peppers, 50

Game hen
   Zucchini-Stuffed Game Hen with Turnip and Mushrooms, 150
Green Coconut Curry with Chicken and Cabbage, 95
Green papaya
   shrimp papaya salad with cashews, 85

Halibut
   Mediterranean halibut in parchment, 137
   Moroccan fish stew, 134
   seafood and butternut squash chowder, 76

Hard-Cooked Eggs with Crab, Avocado and Belgian Endive, 39

Italian Fried Eggs with Sausage and Peppers, 50

Jalapeno
   barbecue sauce, 64
   pork and mango omelet, 43
   seafood and avocado salad, 83
Jicama
   pork ribs with jicama slaw, 143

Kale
   pork tenderloin with cherries and kale, 145

Lamb
   lamb tagine with star anise, 116
   spicy lamb burger with orange herb slaw, 115
Lamb Tagine with Star Anise, 116
Leek
   celery root, leek and pork belly soup, 92
   red snapper with leeks and saffron, 141

wild mushroom soup, 107
Lettuce, romaine
   seafood and avocado salad, 83
Lettuce, spring mix
   turkey with roasted sweet potato, turnip and pear, 103
Lobster
   eggs lobster Oscar with asparagus and cauliflower, 37
   lobster with arugula and spaghetti squash, 129
Lobster with Arugula and Spaghetti Squash, 129

Mango
   pan-seared tuna with caramelized onions and mango salsa, 133
   pork and mango omelet, 43
Mayonnaise, 163
Meatloaf with Roasted Red Pepper and Cauliflower, 117
Mediterranean Halibut in Parchment, 137
Moroccan Fish Stew, 134
Moroccan Spice Blend, 161

Mushrooms
  coddled egg with sun-dried tomatoes and mushrooms, 55
  filet mignon with celery root and mushrooms, 120
  portobello, sausage and egg stack, 47
  sesame shrimp with orange and almonds, 129
  spaghetti squash primavera with chicken, 98
  wild mushroom soup, 107
  zucchini-stuffed game hen with turnip and mushrooms, 150
Mussels
  pan-roasted mussels with onions and basil, 140
Mustard greens
  spicy chicken salad with mustard greens, 93

Pan-Roasted Mussels with Onions and Basil, 140
Pan-Seared Tuna with Caramelized Onions and Mango Salsa, 133

Parsnip
  beet and parsnip chips with shredded chicken, 152
  spicy sweet potato and parsnip soup, 110
Peach
  pork loin chop with peaches, squash and pecans, 144
Pear
  turkey with roasted sweet potato, turnip and pear, 103
Pineapple
  barbecue sauce, 164
Plantain Wraps, 160
  salmon, avocado and pistachio wraps, 35
Porcini mushrooms
  wild mushroom soup, 107
Pork
  pork and mango omelet, 43
  pork belly, 177
  pork loin chop with peaches, squash and pecans, 144
  pork ribs with jicama slaw, 143
  pork tenderloin with cherries and kale, 145
  pork tenderloin with spinach, orange and onions, 89

Pork and Mango Omelet, 43
Pork Belly, 177
Pork belly
  celery root, leek and pork belly soup, pork belly, 177
  Swiss chard, pork belly and bell pepper frittata, 57
Pork Loin Chop with Peaches, Squash and Pecans, 144
Pork Ribs with Jicama Slaw, 143
Pork Tenderloin with Cherries and Kale, 145
Pork Tenderloin with Spinach, Orange and Onions, 89
Pork, baby back ribs
  pork ribs with jicama slaw, 143
Portobello, Sausage and Egg Stack, 47
Pumpkin, Pecan and Coconut Breakfast Bowl, 51

Radish
  bok choy, carrot and radish omelet soup, 62
  chicken salad with carrot, radish and cucumber, 97
Red Snapper with Leeks and Saffron, 141

Roasted Beets with Salmon, Walnuts and Mint, 87
Roasted Eggplant and Cherry Tomatoes with Egg, 59
Roasted Eggplant and Tomato Soup, 109

Salmon
  salmon deviled eggs, 31
  salmon with red cabbage, Brussels sprouts and hazelnuts, 139
  salmon, avocado and pistachio wraps, 35
  salmon, egg and sweet potato pancake, 31
Salmon Deviled Eggs, 41
Salmon with Red Cabbage, Brussels Sprouts and Hazelnuts, 139
Salmon, Avocado and Pistachio Wraps, 35
Salmon, Egg and Sweet Potato Pancake, 31
Sausage
  andouille, 173
  andouille-stuffed tomato, 27
  chorizo, 175
  Italian, 176

Italian fried eggs with sausage and peppers, 50
portobello, sausage and egg stack, 47
sweet potato skin with spinach and Italian sausage, 45
Scrambled Egg Soup with Spinach, 61
Sea Scallops with Cherry Tomatoes, Avocado and Almonds, 131
Seafood and Avocado Salad, 83
Seafood and Butternut Squash Chowder, 76
Sesame Shrimp with Orange and Almonds, 129
Shrimp
  chilled cucumber, avocado and shrimp soup, 79
  seafood and avocado salad, 83
  sesame shrimp with orange and almonds, 129
  shrimp and dill egg custard, 29
  shrimp, red pepper and almond soup, 81
Shrimp and Dill Egg Custard, 29

Shrimp Papaya Salad with Cashews, 85
Shrimp, Red Pepper and Almond Soup, 81
Spaghetti squash
  how to roast, 100
  lobster with arugula and spaghetti squash, 129
  spaghetti squash primavera with chicken, 98
Spaghetti Squash Primavera with Chicken, 98
Spicy Chicken Salad with Mustard Greens, 93
Spicy Lamb Burger with Orange Herb Slaw, 115
Spicy Sweet Potato and Parsnip Soup, 110
Spinach, *see* baby spinach
Steak with Mango, Arugula and Pistachios, 72
Steak, Pepper and Egg with Arugula Pesto, 25
Sweet potato
  spicy sweet potato and parsnip soup, 110
  sweet potato hash with turkey and egg, 67

sweet potato skin with spinach and Italian sausage, 45
turkey with roasted sweet potato, turnip and pear, 103
watercress and sweet potato soup, 105
Sweet Potato Hash with Turkey and Egg, 67
Sweet Potato Skin with Spinach and Italian Sausage
Swiss Chard, Pork Belly and Bell Pepper Frittata, 57

Tangerine
five spice chicken with tangerine and fennel, 146
Tomato(es)
andouille-stuffed tomato, 27
barbecue sauce, 164
coddled egg with sun-dried tomatoes and mushrooms, 55
lamb tagine with star anise, 116
Mediterranean halibut in parchment, 137
Moroccan fish stew, 134

roasted eggplant and tomato soup, 109
sea scallops with cherry tomatoes, avocado and almonds, 131
tuna with poached egg and cherry tomato salsa, 33
veal scallops with cherry tomatoes and celery, 71
Trout with Carrot and Walnuts, 135
Tuna
pan-seared tun with caramelized onions and mango salsa, 133
tuna filet with saffron slaw, 75
tuna with poached egg and cherry tomato salsa, 33
Tuna Filet with Saffron Slaw, 75
Tuna with Poached Egg and Cherry Tomato Salsa, 33
Turkey
turkey with roasted sweet potato, turnip and pear, 103
turkey, zucchini and butternut squash strata, 155

Turkey with Roasted Sweet Potato, Turnip and Pear, 103
Turkey, Cauliflower and Apple Soup, 65
Turkey, Zucchini and Butternut Squash Strata, 155
Turnip
sweet potato hash with turkey and egg, 67
turnip and pear, 103
zucchini-stuffed game hen with turnip and mushrooms, 150
Veal
veal chop with broccoli rabe, 122
veal scallops with cherry tomatoes and celery, 71
Veal Chop with Broccoli Rabe, 122
Veal Scallops with Cherry Tomatoes and Celery, 71
Vegetable Stock, 172

Watercress
roasted beets with salmon, walnuts and mint, 87
watercress and sweet potato soup, 105
Watercress and Sweet Potato Soup, 105

Watermelon, Cucumber and Red Onion with Pork, 91
Wild Mushroom Soup, 107

Yellow squash
pork loin chop with peaches, squash and pecans, 144

Zucchini
andouille-stuffed tomato, 27
curried zucchini spinach soup, 106
Mediterranean halibut in parchment, 137

turkey, zucchini and butternut squash strata, 155
zucchini-stuffed game hen with turnip and mushrooms, 150
Zucchini-Stuffed Game Hen with Turnip and Mushrooms, 150

www.ingramcontent.com/pod-product-compliance
Lightning Source LLC
Chambersburg PA
CBHW071616080526
44588CB00010B/1156